TRANS.

of

HOMOEO DRUG-ENERGY

from

A DISTANCE

DR. B. SAHNI

M.A. (Double), B.T., M.D. (Hom.), F.R.H.A., F.D.R.I.
Director, Research Institute of Sahni Drug Transmission and Homoeopathy
Chief Editor, "Homoeo Tarang" and "The Journal of Homoeo Transmission"
Member, International Homoeopathic League.

B. JAIN PUBLISHERS (P) LTD.

TRANSMISSION OF HOMOEO DRUG-ENERGY FROM A DISTANCE

First edition: 1970

2nd Revised & enlarged edition: 1978

3rd Revised & enlarged edition: 1993

Reprint edition: 2000, Jan. 2005

Price: Rs. 99.00

Published by Kuldeep Jain for

B. Jain Publishers (P) Ltd.

1921, Street No. 10, Chuna Mandi, Paharganj, New Delhi 110 055 (INDIA)
Phones: 2358 0800, 2358 1100, 2358 1300
Fax: 011-2358 0471; *Email:* bjain@vsnl.com
Website: www.bjainbooks.com

Printed in India by

J.J. Offset Printers

522, FIE, Patpar Ganj, Delhi - 110 092
Phones: 2216 9633, 2215 6128

ISBN: 81-7021-135-2

BOOK CODE: BS-2457

DEDICATED
TO
LOVERS OF SCIENCE

CONTENTS

PART ONE

Some Researches

PART TWO

Transmission of Drug-Energy Through Detached Hair of Patient.

Dr. Jugal Kishore   Resi. 86, Golf Links
B.Sc., D.M.S., M.D. (Hom.)   New Delhi-110003
Hony. Physician to the President of India
Hony. Advisor to the Govt. of India
President, Central Council of Homoeopathy

FOREWORD

I have been asked to write a Foreword to the Second Edition of Dr. B. Sahni's book, 'Transmission of Homoeo Drug Energy from a Distance'. I know Dr. Sahni more intimately through patients who have been benefited by his treatment. He has been a tireless worker for the advancement of science and art of Homoeopathy. I must, however, express my ignorance about his theories and techniques of transmission of drug energy from a distance. The very fact that many people claim that they have been affected from a considerable distance by drug energy where their hair was immersed in the potentised drug needed by them, arouses one's curiosity regarding the explanation of the phenomenon.

The author has cited numerous cases, some very difficult indeed. It is, therefore, desirable that these phenomena should be examined by a team consisting of Homoeopathic Clinicians and Physicists. The transmission of energy is claimed through contact, through a specimen of blood, through hair by contact with the indicated drug. The most fantastic claim has been made through the contact of the indicated remedy with signature of the person. The author claims that a number of experiments have been successful. Similarly during telephonic conversation with the patients, the author experienced effect of the drug when the bottle containing the appropriate drug was opened.

Apparently, the author has travelled much beyond Hahnemann when the latter advocated transmission of drug energy olfaction.

The author has tried to explain that the drug energy is transmitted through 'Electro-magnetic waves'. These assumptions, however, have been made on theoretical grounds. Nature of drug energy of Homoeopathic medicine is still an unknown entity; its physical properties are unknown; at least, no scientific instrument has so far been invented to sense it. I think that Homoeopathic drug in potencies has a special bio-physical energy of its own which triggers specially nerve centre in the brain to mobilise the curative reactions.

Anyway, the experiences of Dr. Sahni are exciting enough and I feel that we should first observe the phenomena and duplicate the results as claimed by Dr. Sahni, before we try to offer scientific explanations.

I, therefore, recommend the Homoeopathic scientists to explore the uncharted seas in company with Dr. Sahni and verify his 'discoveries'. The journey can be exciting enough.

Jugal Kishore

FOREWORD TO 1st EDITION

There are more things in heaven and earth
than are dreamt of in your philosophy.

- Shakespeare

Here is a book of an unusual type which seeks to explore
uncharted territory. The exploration of the unknown is a
fascinating subject. A special type of mental make-up is necessary for research of this type. One has to discard all preconceived notions and ideas. The orthodox scientist or the
academician would be inclined to reject outright the thesis of
this book. As a matter of fact, when I questioned a number of
qualified homeopaths, before whom a demonstration of transmission of drug-energy to patients, was given were either
sceptical or down-right hostile. An attitude of this kind is hardly
conducive to unravelling the secrets of nature. One has to
cultivate an open and receptive mind to understand the theory
and practice of this new system of transmission of drug-energy.

Dr. Sahni's transmission of drug-energy through the
patients' hair depends upon radiesthesia. Dowsing or water
divining which is based on radiesthesia has been practised since
time immemorial. It is only of late that some scientists have
turned their attention to the scientific study of dowsing. A few
scientists here and there have also been experimenting with
medical radiesthesia or the transmission of energy of drugs over
distances. Some of the notable names in this line of research are
Walter De La Wethered and late Dr. B. Bhattacharya of Naihati,
West Bengal. I believe the most advanced research in this line
has been done by Dr. Bhattacharya, who has had very interesting results in what he calls "Cosmic Ray Therapy". However,
the credit for large-scale experiments in the transmission of
homoeopathic drugs over long distances must go to the author
of this book. He has used this system extensively in his
therapeutic work with excellent results. The discovery of Dr. B.

Sahni has nothing to do with telepathy or spiritual healing. In these days of radio and television, it should not be difficult to believe that the energy of potentised drugs can be transmitted over long distances. If wireless waves can be beamed to distant planets, it should be theoretically possible to transmit the energy of drugs in the shape of radiations. The hair of the patient acts as an aerial to broadcast the drug-energy. The hair is in rapport with the patient and serves as a link with the patient wherever he may be.

This book is a pioneering effort in a new line which is practically unknown in India. I am sure, it will stimulate research not only in the medical field but for other purposes as well.

New Delhi
12.5.70

K.L. Bhola
Dy. Director General
(P. & T.), New Delhi.

x

I have spent a full day learning about Dr. Sahni's experiments and achievements in the area of Homoeopathic hair transmission and am very excited about the possibilities for such treatment. I see application in many areas including Criminology, mental health treatment, drug rehabilitation as well as treatment of physical and mental symptoms in man and animals. I truly hope the important discoveries made here will one day be known and utilized to the extent it deserves.

Richard Kass
35 Mc. Commik Sene,
Atherton, California
U.S.A. 94025
Participant on Berkeley professional Studies Programme in India in health and Medical Science from university of California Berkeley.

Dr. Amar Chandra Jha, M.Sc., Ph. D.
Department of Chemistry,
B.N. College, Patna & a Homoeopath

I have gone through Dr. B. Sahni's book entitled "TRANS-MISSION OF HOMOEO DRUG ENERGY FROM A DISTANCE". Author's new method of homoeopathic treatment attracted me at the first glance but I wanted to ascertain the facts by direct experimentation. Hence I followed his method in case of a number of patients suffering from fever, cold and cough, wounds, abscess, croup, various troubles of mouth, rheumatism, liver troubles, diarrhoea, dysentery, troubles of worm, blood pressure, eczema, various injuries etc. & all the patients were speedily cured by transmission of appropriate remedy. Whenever transmission using a particular drug and potency could not affect the cure, I also tested the oral method of administration of the same drug in the same potency which also could not cure. For cure of a patient, appropriate remedy and potency-both are required, no matter whether Sahni's method of transmission or oral method of administration of drug is followed. I have not even the slightest doubt about the success of this process of transmission of homoeo drug energy from a distance.

Further, the problem is to offer a satisfactory explanation of the observed phenomena. In this direction also an attempt has been made under the chapter, "The principle involved in transmission of homoeo drug energy from a distance or mechanism of transmission".

It is needless to say that this is a well written book containing the details of a number of difficult cases cured by transmission process. The author has also included some cases cured by other homoeopaths working on this line. This clearly shows that homoeopathic world is accepting Sahni's ideas regarding transmission of homoeo drug energy. For full acquaintance with this new discovery, every homoeopath must have a copy of this book in his possession. The homoeopathic world is proud of Dr. Sahni. I wish him success in life.

A.C. Jha.

Dr. S.V. SOHONI, *I.C.S.*
LOKAYUKTA

4, Kautliya Marga,
PATNA-800001
"BIHAR STATE"
Dated 9.1.1975

Dr. Bandhu Sahni's work, "Transmission of homoeo drug energy from a distance" is thought-provoking contribution to theory and practice of homoeopathic science. Even the most skeptical mind would not be able to resist his claim that the conclusions set forth in this book were based on scientific method as applied to a number of experiments conducted by the author. While Dr. Sahni's analysis might recall ancient Indian speculation about transmission of energy in space, its partial endorsement by a practitioner of homoeopathy like him was totally unexpected.

One may hope that the learned author would be able to marshal even a larger body of facts to enable the common lay man to appreciate the possibilities of science even better, for promoting relief to suffering humanity.

S.V. Sohoni

Dr. D. Mandal M.Sc., Ph.D., D. Phil.
Reader in Chemistry,
Patna University,
Patna-5
26.9.1977

"Transmission of Homoeo Drug Energy from a Distance" Written by Dr. Bandhu Sahni is the study of a new method of treatment under Homoeopathic system. Drug is applied on the patient's hair and the patient gets the healing effect at a distance.

Shall I call in analog-to-analog transmission of Bioplasma? Whether the intraorganism connections not linearly connecting the stimulated acupuncture point (in this method a hair) by way of Classical nervous system affect a vital organ in the part of the body of the patient ?

Whatever be the reason Dr. Sahni believes after experimental observations that the drugs work and the transmission from a distance operates. This may be parapsychological phenomenon, which has been believed to exist by the Russians who are seeking practical applications & so is Dr. Sahni seriously inquisitive to prove the phenomenon.

Characteristics of acupuncture points during conditions of well being, ill health emotional and mental stimulations during the course of the treatment shown through Kirlian photography might be of immensely valuable scientific information. Life force has been talked since centuries but it is Kirlian Photography and other forms of scientific researches which are being carried on in Russia, which would make it visible to all. Americans are still trying to prove the existance of extra-sensory perception.

I hope, the technique based on Homoeopathic system in the hands of Dr. Sahni will prove of considerable utility in the healing of millions and millions of poor people of India and his search for the new and cultivation of the hidden will be thus immensely rewarded. The foundation theory of Homoeopathic treatment : Similia Similibus Curenter, has not remained just a passing phrase. It has influenced the social, political and even scientific laws. Dr. Sahni, by pursuing the method would do immense good in healing the ailments of suffering humanities in India and abroad.

Conclusively, I do hope that the technique would prove scientifically to be operative so that it may be applied in Chemotherapy and Radiotherapy as well and other difficult diseases like cancer may be treated successfully.

D.Mandal

V.V. N A T H E N, I.A.S.
COMMISSIONER OF MINES &
GEOLOGY, GOVT. OF BIHAR

P A T N A
The 29th September, 1977

Dr. Bandhu Sahni has been doing pioneering work in field of healing for the past few years. He has for some years now experimenting with the healing by drug transmission over distance. Despite the limited resources at his disposal for experimental work, he has kept regular record of his work and results. His main handicap has been the lack of an institutional base and research facilities with qualified workers, so that those could be effective documentation of results obtained.

Results of known cases of cures claimed are remarkable. He requires assistance on a large scale to establish his results on regular scientific documentation to bring it upto standards of acceptable basis.

The prospect before Dr. Sahni is very exciting. I hope that suffering humanity would be able to draw succour more and more from his ministrations.

V.V. NATHEN

Dr. Ram Swaroop Sinha
G.B.V.C., P.G., D.T.V. Sc.
P.G. (Australia) M.D.E.H.
Joint Director, Animal Husbandry,
Govt. of Bihar, Patna

I have the privilege to know Dr. Bandhu Sahni as an outstanding physician in the field of Homoeopathy. His thrilling new discovery of "Homoeo Drug Energy Transmission from a Distance" based on electro-magnetic waves appears to be similar to the well known "*Raman Effect*", as in the latter case, light of definite frequency is incident on the substance while in the former case, the whole range of electromagnetic waves, is claimed to be incident on the transmitting set. His theory, based on innumerable experimental observations, seems to have revolutionised the Homoeo-Science, and works like a space-conqueror in Homoeopathy.

That, he has been taking keen interest even in his busy hours, in extending this dynamic method of simple, cheap, and effective cure to Veterinary ailments also, shows a Scientist's continued gracious approach to solve the immense problems in the field of Animal Science too with a view to better the lot of the farmers.

I am sure, the second edition of his valuable book entitled, "Transmission of Homoeo Drug Energy from a Distance (A new Discovery), will continue to prove a boon to the suffering humanity and the dumb millions.

Ram, Swaroop Sinha
26.9.77

Dr. Kailash Singh,
M.B.B.S., M.D., (DERM)
Asstt. Professor (Skin & V.D.)
Rajendra Medical College, Ranchi-9

The recent discovery of "TRANSMISSION OF HOMOEO DRUG ENERGY FROM A DISTANCE" by Dr. Bandhu Sahni explained in this book is the result of very careful and tiring investigation on purely scientific lines based on Bio-Physics and Bio-Chemistry. His theory of drug transmission from a distance has been well supported by experiments and tests on patients of various categories including patients of incurable diseases like Cancer, Azospermia etc. I have myself tried his method of Homoeo Drug Transmission through hair on many patients including specialists of the Modern Medical science and found it most effective and quick in action. Dr. Sahni by his unique discovery has proved beyond doubt Dr. S. Hahnemann's "Similia Similibus Curenter" through Similia from a distance. His discovery, I believe is far ahead the time. His method of drug Transmission is quicker and safer in use. It needs wide publicity for proper understanding and utility. To him belongs the honour of making this discovery a land mark in the History of Homoeopathic Medical Science.

Dr. SHREENIVAS, 22.7.70
Professor & Head of Department of Medicine,
P.W. Medical College, and Head of
Department of Cardiovascular Diseases,
Medical College & Hospital,
Patna.

Homoeopathy is not a hoax. And the homoeopath is not a humbug. That sometimes homoeopathy scores over the other systems of medical treatment is a fact. It has the additional advantages of being cheap and least bothersome for the patient. The theoretical conceptions on which homoeopathy is based are queer and strange. They are inexplicable. Nevertheless the drugs seem to act.

Dr. B. Sahni, the author of this book, "Transmission of Homoeo Drug-Energy from A Distance (A New Discovery)", is a renowned homoeopath and is credited with having cured many "difficult" cases. He has now invented a new method or technique for achieving his ends. He procures a hair from the body of his patient. The suitable and properly selected homoeopathic medicine is brought in contact with the hair and it is claimed that the effect of the medicine becomes manifest on the patient and his disease, irrespective of the distance separating the patient and his hair. It seems to be a case of treatment by proxy.

It is propounded that the hair works like the antenna of a broadcasting station and the contact with the patient is established through some unknown and mysterious power of the ionised homoeopathic medicine which, after the considerable dilutions, acquires a power and potentiality unique of its own kind. It is conjectured that the transmission of this effectiveness may be akin or similar to the transmission of thought waves or of the electromagnetic waves. The author has no claims to having discovered the way it really works but he is sure that it does work. In this approach of the author there is nothing unscientific. His findings and results will have to be statistically analyzed.

The mysteries of nautre can only be unravelled by scientific experimentations.

I have no personal knowledge of the effectiveness of this kind of treatment but it is fascinating to think of such possibilities. It should not be discarded without reason. Many hypotheses were scoffed and jeered at before they were found to be correct.

Dr. Sahni's enthusiasm for scientific investigations has compelled me to write these few lines of appreciation. I wish him a grand success in his endeavour. The phenomenon described by him may usher in a great discovery. It requires to be tested and verified. His zeal is contagious.

Shreenivas

N.B. : *Opinion on the first edition of this book.*

SHAKTI NIVAS

Boring Road, Patna

Dated 14.6.1970

Phuldeo Sahay Varma,

M.Sc., A.I.I.Sc..

EX-UNIVERSITY PROFESSOR AND PRINCIPAL
COLLEGE OF TECHNOLOGY AND EX-DEAN
OF THE FACULTIES OF SCIENCE
AND OF TECHNOLOGY
BANARAS HINDU
UNIVRSITY
EX-INSPECTOR OF COLLEGES, BIHAR UNIVERSITY.
EX-EDITOR, HINDI ENCYCLOPEDIA. GOVT. OF INDIA.

I have gone through some pages of the printed forms of a small book, entitled, "TRANSMISSION OF HOMOEO DRUG-ENERGY FROM A DISTANCE (A NEW DISCOVERY)" by Dr. B. Sahni.

I have found the reading interesting. The author has developed a new system of treatment by Homoeopathic drugs and has cited some examples of successful cure by his new method.

The explanation of the effectiveness of drugs seems to be plausible.

I wish the author success in his enterprise.

P.S. Varma

N.B.- Opinion on the first edition of this book.

all India Magic Circle
आल इंडिया मैजिक सर्किल
276-1, RASH BEHARY AVENUE,
CALCUTTA-19 (INDIA)

ALL INDIA MAGIC CIRCLE
PATNA BRANCH

President :-
(3578) B.P. BARANWAL,
WIZARD—"BURNOL"
B.A., B.L., I.N.S. (Paris)
Magistrate, (Bihar Civil Service)
Raj Banshi Nagar, Road No.1,
Patna-1.

National President :-
(Padmashri) P.C. SORCAR F.R.
A.S. (Lond.), J.P. "Indrajal"
Calcutta-19. (India

Dr. B. Sahni's novel approach to medicine and treatment is more miraculous than magic, is more effective and quick in action than mantras.

I have myself seen the wonderful action of this 'wizard' of Homoeopathic world. His commendable discovery of "Transmission of Homoeopathic drug-energy" has surpassed all others in the arena of medical therapy. It is a wonderful 'augury' in Homoeopthic science.

I wish him continued strength and success in this field for the betterment of sufferings of down trodden and ailing mankind.

B.P. Baranwal.
15.6.1970

N.B.- Opinion on the first edition of this book.

ACKNOWLEDGEMENTS

The author expresses his thankfulness to Mr. A. Kumar of Bhagalpur who offered himself for the first experiment. He is very much grateful to Dr. Chandra Prakash, the Ex-editor of the, "Torch of Homoeopathy", Jaipur who encouraged him by giving an editorial note with valuable suggestions and appreciation on his first article on "Transmission of Homoeopathic Drug-Energy." He offers his thanks to Dr. Diwan Harishchand, Dr. B.P. Gyani, Dr. P.L. Shrivastava, Dr. Sachchidanand, Sri P.K. Sinha, Dr. Bechan, Dr.S.N. Prasad, Dr. K.L. Mishra, Prof. M.S. Shrivastava & Prof. T.R.C. Sinha for kind help and valuable suggestions. His thanks are overdue to Dr. N.K. Sinha, Dr. N.K.P. Sinha, Dr. D.N. Pathak, Dr. R.N. Singh, Dr. H.S. Verma, Dr. K.N. Sinha, Dr. S.P. Mehrotra, Dr. N. Mandal & many others who experimented his discovery and encouraged him.

He confesses his indebtedness to Prof. R.C. Singh. Deptt. of Physics, M.J.K. College Bettiah & Dr. K.N. Lal for translating his ideas into scientific language. He owes indebtedness to Dr. D.C. Kern for his kind co-operation and giving opportunity for demonstration and lecture on the occasion of annual function of Bihar State Homoeopathic Congress of All India Institute of Homoeopathy. He is thankful to Dr. B. Prasad of Gaya for the same and sending a report of demonstration and experimenting the discovery.

He offers his deep gratefulness to Dr. B.N. Saksena for his open-mindedness, co-operation, experimenting, encouraging and accepting the superiority of "Transmission..." over his own discovery, "Radiation of Plants & Herbs from a Distance-Psycho-Medico-Therapy." He cannot remain silent without giving thanks to Dr. K.P. Shrivastava who reported some of his clinical observations by "Transmission." and Mrs. K. Sinha for her co-operation. He is thankful to Dr. S.N. Mishra, Dr. N.K. Mishra, Dr. L.P. Singh, Dr. M.L. Choudhary and Shri D.M. Prasad for their help in typing work and seeing proofs.

He is very much grateful to Dr. S. Nath & Sri B.K.P. Verma for their kind co-operation and suggestions. He is very much thankful to his wife, Dr. S. Sahni and his son, Dr. M.K.

Sahni without whose help this could not be completed. He is very much indebted to Sahni Homoeo Pharmacy & Publication for publishing this book. He is thankful to Bharati Press, Tarang Press & Publication for printing 1st & 2nd edition respectively and Sri Ram Ekbal Matho, Rekha Binding House for Binding works.

The author expresses his deep gratitude to Mr. V.P. Kashyap I.A.S. Health Commissioner, Bihar for giving opportunity to experiment the theory on all the members of his family. He will remain ever thankful to Mr. K.L. Bhola for his keen interest, writing foreward, co-operation and valuable suggestions. He is very much thankful to Dr. V.L. Shrivastava who encouraged him by his bitter criticism in the very inception of the discovery, resulting in a still better stamina to justify the theory of "Transmission."

He is thankful to Mr. B. Prasad for writing "About the Author," Mrs. Prasad, Dr. P. Choudhary, Dr. R.N. Sinha & Sri S.N. Singh for their co-operation and encouragement. He is not less thankful to Dr. S.K. Verma and Dr. (Mrs.) Verma for their co-operation.

The author extends his thanks to the Rupa Studio, Shri M.B. Parimal, the Hind Art College, Sri Anandi Pd. Badal, Miss Manju and Sri N. Nirava for Photography, Block-making & artistic portrait.

The author is very grateful to Sri P.S. Verma who kindly went through some pages of the manuscipt of the book and gave his learned opinion on plausibility of "Transmission." He extends his hearty thanks to Sri B.P. Barnwal, President, All India Magic Circle for his kind perusal of the manuscript of the book and his expression of appreciation after keenly observing the magical effects of this discovery.

Thanks are due to all those who helped him in bringing out the present volume.

The author is indebted to authors particularly Dr. P. Sankaran, Dr. B. Bhattacharya and Mr. Peter Tompkins and Mr. Christopher Bird, whose works have been consulted and quoted liberally.

The author is very thankful to Dr. S.V. Sohoni and Sri V.V. Nathen for their kind expressions of appreciations and encouragement.

xxiv

He will remain ever thankful to Dr. Jugal Kishore for sparing valuable time from his busy hours to grace this book with his foreword and precious suggestions. He expresses his thanks to Dr. Meredith Lowry and Master Richard Kass, U.S.A. for their keen interest in this method & co-operation in furthering this discovery.

Thanks are due to Dr. Bishwanath Prasad, Dr. Bindeshwar Prasad, Dr. P. Sah, Dr. R.K.P. Sinha for their co-operation in preparing the manuscript and giving their experimental observations for inclusion in the book and reading proof etc.

Thanks to Sri J. Sahni, Sri K. Thakur, and Sri R. Singh, Homoeo students for helping in preparing manuscript.

The author is very thankful to Dr. Kailash Singh for his expression of appreciation.

He is thankful to Dr. J.N. Kanjilal who rendered his help by giving comments on the first edition about ionisation of drugs which led to the present theory.

The author is very thankful to Dr. A.C. Jha for experimenting this method and rendering help in explaining the mechanism of this discovery and seeing proofs.

He is thankful to Dr. K. Prasad, Principal U.H. Medical College and Hospital, for his kind appreciation.

He is thankful to Dr. G.L. Joneja, Sri B. Prasad Director and Sri K.K. Prasad Asstt. Prof. English Institute, Bihar, Patna, and Sri S.D. Singh, Lecturer, State Institute of Education, Bihar, Patna, for their help in seeing and correcting the manuscript.

He is thankful to Sri Mahadev Behari, Sri P.C. Singh, Smt. P. Verma for their help in seeing proofs.

He is very grateful to Reverend Swami Hansanand of Coimbatore for experimenting and sending observations and giving encouragement from time to time.

He is thankful to Dr. Ram Swaroop Sinha for his cooperation in the veterinary field and his words of appreciation.

Thanks to master Pradeep Kr. Sahni and M.K. Sahni for their hard labour in publishing this.

EXORDIUM TO THE SECOND EDITION

Under the pressure of great demand for the book which is out of print now, the author was requested by the publisher to write its 2nd edition to satisfy the curiosity of the physician as well as the lovers of science. The importance of this edition lies in the evolution of theory on Transmission of Drug Energy from a distance and experimental observations of cures of so called incurable diseases like Cancer, Azospermia etc. and inclusion of some more topics. In the beginning the phenomenon was explained by citing examples of scorpion or snake-bites and Alsatian dog.

These analogies do not seem correct and appealing hence another field was hunted out. An attempt was made to offer a scientific explanation of the process of transmission of Homoeo drug energy with the idea of "IONISATION". The homoeopathic potentised drug is nothing but energy in ionised form. When a medicated glouble is dissolved in a phial, it makes its field in the phial. When this field comes in contact with the field of the hair the resultant field becomes so intense & rapid that it begins to radiate energy waves, or pulses at a particular frequency. As the constitution & vibratory state of the hair which transmits the resultant energy (effect of medicine) is the same as that of the body from which the hair was detached (patient). This vibration of hair caused by the effect of medicine causes a similar & sympathetic vibration in the body. The propagation of vibration of the effect or drug does not require actual physical contact of drug with the body as it is only the energy of drug which is transmitted in a similar way as that of Radio or Television.

The above explanation as to how medicine energy is transmitted to the patient at a distance through detached hair is not sound because the theory of ionisation may not be equally applicable in case of all the Homoeo drugs obtained from various sources.

Efforts were made to find out the general explanation and ultimately a new idea of transmission based in emission of electromagnetic waves from Homoeo drugs has been developed which is discussed in detail in chapter VI of part II under the "Mechanism of Drug Transmission". In the new mechanism it is assumed that omnipresent electromagnetic waves are incident on the medicine (Solid or liquid) at infinite number of planes and infinite number of beams scatter in all directions at right angles to the direction of incidence. This is very similar to the well known "Raman Effect". The hair or any natural belonging placed in the field of medicine assumes the frequency of the scattered beams and transmits this medicinal energy to the patient with the velocity of light & thus the patient at a distance is influenced by the medicinal energy instantaneously.

With the development of this very idea, it is crystal clear now that :—

(1)   Distance is no bar. This hypothesis is a reality now.

(2)   All the potencies are operative for any distance. Due to hasty generalisation and malobservations it was written in the first edition that the higher potency covers greater distance. Successful transmission of drug energy using medicine only of potency 200 from Patna to Delhi. Amritsar, U.S.A. etc. confirms this very idea.

(3)   Any natural belonging to the patient may be used for transmitting medicine energy. Experiments on blood, sputum, photograph, signature, voice (in Telephone & Taperecorder) etc. along with hair have been made successfully on patients. The same principle as applied in case of hair works here too.

Some chapters have been rewritten and some additions or ommissions have been made here & there

(a)   A new chapter "Acupuncture, zone therapy and Yoga" has been included.

(b)   The principle involved in transmission of drug has been rewritten.

(c)   Mode of action of Homoeo dilution is still controversial. An attempt has been made to sum up the various ideas concerning the action of various attenuations, which has been included in the chapter, "The drug and potency."

(d)   The chapter "Experimental observations" have been rewritten. A number of difficult cases & so called incurable cases like AZOSPERMIA, CANCER, DIABETES etc. has been included under different headings.

The chapter "COSMIC RAY THERAPY" has been renamed as "TREATMENT THROUGH PHOTOGRAPH". Some more experiments done in the field of agriculture by others and in Homoeopathy by the author have been added. Some alterations in the titles of some chapters have been made and some more topics were added in different chapters.

A few words about use of hair are necessary. There is no need of uprooting the hair from the head. It may be cut from any part of the body not essentially the head. Hair was taken from St. Vinoba's chest, and it was cut from the axilla of Sri Sri Jagatguru Shankaracharya of Puri and medicine was transmitted successfully.

B. Sahni

EXORDIUM TO THE FIRST EDITION

After all what is the summum bonum of life? Is it amassing wealth or obtaining health or wisdom, or attaining liberation? Why is there unrest in the bosom of human beings? Is the man possessing vast wealth happy? If so, why then further craving? What is the reason behind it that he is not happy? Man is made not only of matter, life and mind. If it be so, he should have been happy with the vast wealth and mundane power, but it is not so. He has something transcendental in him. He possesses a spark of Divine Light which is clouded by ignorance. He is a rational animal. His animality may be satisfied with sensual pleasures in the material possessions but his rationality and spirituality must demand something immaterial. The material possessions cannot satisfy the immaterial or spiritual entity in man. That is why man is not happy. Then what will make him happy? Attainment of Sachidanand—Consciousness—Existence—Bliss who is omniscient, omnipotent and omnipresent, may be the summum bonum of life.

Man, being born on earth will have to face decay and death even though to the maximum he can avoid pains and miseries, but that ideal health is difficult in the existing order. Our life on earth is a mixture of joys and sorrows. Our philosophy starts with pessimism and ends in optimism, full of vigour and enlightenment. Miseries befall man but he, being intelligent, strives to find out the remedies to end them. Different approaches have been made to get rid of them. There are philosophical as well as therapeutic ways to overcome. Formerly the philosophers were the custodians of health and spirit, body and mind. The puzzle of body, life, mind and soul has been confronting us from time immemorial. The materialist gives emphasis on the material aspect while the idealist on the spiritual aspect, but problem remains unsolved. In course of time medical science appeared to take charge of the former from the philosophers leaving the latter to them, but it made the man mechanical having no regard for spirit or vital force. Dr. S. Hahnemann, the father of Homoeopathy, putting his firm feet on the ground and head in the heaven, made the medical science a meeting ground of

Physical Science and Metaphysics. he treated the man as a whole possessing body, life, mind and spirit and gave an immortal principle of Similia Similibus Curenter to the world for suffering humanity, which is a Divine Art of Healing—a combination of science and philosophy. He saw the latent energy hidden in the tiny globule of Homoeopathic dynamic medicine which reminds me of Prakriti of the Sankhya system of Metaphysics. Every thing of the universe is an effect of some cause. Every effect has material as well as efficient cause. Prakriti is the material cause of the manifested universe as well as its efficient cause. Prakriti is the ultimate cause of the world of objects. After destruction of objects physical elements are resolved into atoms, the atoms into energy and so on, till all products are resolved into the unmanifested, eternal Prakriti. Prakriti is constituted by three gunas of sattva (Neutrons), rajas (Electrons) and tamas (protons). The three gunas preponderate over each other when there is a tremendous commotion in the infinite womb of Prakriti by very presence of Purusa. Out of disturbance of equilibrium or chaos there is cosmos. Every thing of the universe evolves from the unfathomable womb of Prakriti. This topic concerns Metaphysics hence unwillingly I have to twist my course to the physical science as I do not want to be lost in its puzzle but it can be said that to attain the summum bonum of life sound health is essential. If we go on breaking, dividing, and subdividing matter, we will reach a stage where our reason feels staggered in its attempt to grasp its real nature. Scientists come to give nomenclature of atoms, electrons, protons, neutrons, positrons etc. which along with the universe remain like appearance of Bradley of the West and Maya of the Advaita Vedanta (Monism). Thus matter becomes energy and energy matter. The subtle energy gives dimensions to every object which is perceptual to our senses. It is invisible. X-Ray and Laser Ray can penetrate or make a hole in a diamond but it is not visible. Ultrasonic sound, Infra-red waves etc. can penetrate the body but neither the person nor the operator can see it.

Let us cast a glance over the Homoeopathic medicine. What really is Homoeopathic potentized drug? Is it a latent energy hidden in the matter which is derived by breaking, dividing, and subdividing the medicinal substance. By the process of subdividing we get to an electronic stage or even beyond that where our imagination too feels staggered. It may be that by so doing we reach the substratum (Prakriti). There we may have glimpse of Divine sparks. There is no distinction between the space occupied by the house after its destruction and the eternal space where we are lost.

For practical purposes we have to halt at the electronic stage only where the physical science has reached to-day so that the explanation of the Homoeopathic potentized drug may be grasped by the scientific discipline. The modern science cannot explain the existence and activities of the potencies like C.M.D.M., C.M.M. etc. That is why I beg apology from my brother Homoeopaths to excuse me for coming down to the potentized drug in the form of "IONS" which may appeal to the scientific world.

Meditation on the subtle nature of Homoeo Drug reveals that it is beyond chemical and physical laws. On this point Hahnemann himself says that potentised medicines "are no longer subject to chemical laws." We know that phosphorus oxidises when exposed to air. Further Hahnemann points out, "A powder of phosphorus in highest potency may remain in a desk, without losing its medicinal properties or even changing into phosphoric acid. He adds, "A remedy which has been elevated to the highest potency.....is no longer, subject to the laws of neutralization". Dr. Tyler remarks, "If this were not the case how could we carry about our little phials of medicated globules, secure in knowledge that they would not interfere with one another, or neutralize one another, but would be always remedy for use, and never fail us provided they are correctly prescribed."

How could the subtle energy or potentized drug be neutralized by the gross smell, smoke, tobacco etc. was the problem in the beginning of my studies and practice? I had to cogitate on this. My reason was or is never satisfied with the traditional notion, beliefs, and ritual of so many Don'ts of teachers and physicians of great acumen of the past and the present. My simple logic is that the subtle cannot be neutralized by the gross like smoke, smell, tobacco etc. I began to administer medicines to the patients while smoking or chewing betel with tobacco, using onion, garlic etc. but the action of the drugs could not be neutralized or hampered by these. As soon as the tiny globule saturated with potentized drug was put on the tongue full of the betel with tobacco of an officer, suffering from actue pain in his rectum due to piles, his agonising pain vanished like magic. The smoking patients having a tiny globule were benefited. In this way I have observed prompt action of drugs in innumerable cases while using many Dont's." It does not mean that I do not believe in purity and antidotes and I do advocate smoking etc. Purity must be maintained but we should not be so dogmatic. The dogma of "Don'ts" reminds me of an episode of a cased cat and marriage-ceremony. In the past at the time of marriage-ceremony, the domestic cat used to spoil milk, curd, etc. The old lady of the house to avoid this nuisance got the cat encased by putting a basket over it. A newly married bride was observing this through her Ghunghat. When she became mother and marriage-ceremony was to be performed in her house, she also got a cat encased in the above manner on that auspicous occasion and henceforward encasing a cat on such occasion became a custom. So is the case in our practice of Homoeopathy. So many drosses have cropped in. We do not exercise our god-gifted reason. The dogmatic "Don'ts" have sprung from the maintenance of purity at the time of proving drugs. The exciting factors were kept aloof from the subjects at the time of proving so that confusion might not arise regarding effects.

The existing tradition and practice of orthodox school have left their stamps on the use of doses. It is a wonder how a great doctor and thinker like C. Hering M.D. used to prescribe one globule for infants and 4 or 5 for adults! In the modern school of medical therapy quantity of doses due to predominance of matter in drug plays a vital part. Large dose of Arsenic may take life of a patient but potentized Arsenic according to similimum even in a dozen globules dose will not do so. Quality plays an important role in our practice, hence the questions of difference in no. of globules for infants and adults should not arise. Will 5 globules of potentized Arsenic do any harm to infants and one globule or part of it be inadequate to stimulate the economy of an adult? Is this practice not dogmatic? What will be the qualitative value of one and five globules? Where is the principle of minimum dose? Why not to follow the minimum possible dose of S. Hahnemann equally for infants and adults? Potency may be considered for age-group or conditions of the patients.

What a tremendous energy of electro-magnetic type stored in a tiny globule of medicine? Why will it not affect the person handling it? Why will it not affect through olfactory or tactual organs? Why will the phial containing medicine, if opened not influence the persons sitting all around in the chamber? Those, who believe that they will not affect, have not imbibed the very spirit of Homoeopathy. They are sceptical in their practice! They have no faith in subtlety of drug!

The discovery of Radio and Television should have opened our inward eyes. Radio waves, electro-magnetic waves, ultra-violet and Infra-red waves, light, colour and sound waves, Roentgen rays, supersonic waves, cosmic rays and even thought waves in case of telepathy can be transmitted. The space craft can be controlled from the earth in its way to moon and return journey, then why not subtle energy of Homoeopathic medicine can be transmitted ? That was the problem which had been taxing my brain. The past and the existing events, and phenomena of nature nurture the seed of any new discovery. Why did the person, carrying Aesculus in his pocket for his ailing relative, get rid of his haemorrhoids ? Is this phenomenon not sufficient to give a clue to a new discovery? It should have been done long-long ago after this event. However, the subtle nature of dynamic Homoeo drug let me cogitate to find out the medium through which the drug energy may be channelised. I made an enquiry from Dr. Boyd, M.B.B.S., M.R.C.P. Glassgow about the Emenometer invented by his late learned father. From his letter it transpires that it was not successful. It is only for research purpose. It came to my mind that the mightiest machine of to-day cannot control the activity of dynamic drug and I went on my mission. One day, in the night of 5.1.1967 it came to my mind all of a sudden that some natural belonging to the patient may give some clue for "Transmission". It was a restless night for me. In the morning of 6.1.1967 all on a sudden I requested Sri Kumar who had colic pain due to peptic ulcer to give me one hair from his head. I put that hair on paper on the table and Alb. 200 one globule was brought in contact with the root of that hair. It acted miracle. He felt a churning sensation within his abdomen. Then the hair was detached from the medicine and his pain was reduced by 75%. At once it stroke to me! It might be a psychological effect on the mind of the patient. I told Sri Kumar that the remaining 25% pain will go this time and I poured one drop of Ars. Alb. 30 on the root of that hair. His pain became so intense that he left my chamber in agony. My joy knew no bounds and I began to experiment on that line with success. I wrote down one article, under the caption, "The

Homoeo. Dynamic Medicine can be transmitted" which was published in the "Torch of Homoeopathy, Jaipur, Rajasthan, with encouraging editorial notes by Dr. Chandra Prakash in the April 1967 issue. I began to preach this discovery among friends, disciples and others. Queries began to pour on this discovery and I tried my best to reply them as far as practicable. Articles on experimental observations were published in different Homoeopathic journals. Efforts were made to collect literature on recent researches in the field of Homoeopathy as well as in others. The theory of "Transmission" is supported by other researches like "electro-magnetic waves" of human body by Dr. Abrams of San Francisco, "Emenometer" by Dr. Boyd of Glassgow, "Pulse Rate Theory", Medical Radiesthesia", "The Cosmic Rays Therapy", Dynamic action of drugs and plants" etc.

Formerly in articles and discussions I used to explain the theory of "Transmission" by giving analogies of a detective dog, scorpion and snake—bites but now after constant efforts scientific explanation has been found out which may satisfy the curiosity of lovers of science. If this will not fulfil the scientific discipline I may be excused for encroaching the field.

I may submit that the action of "Transmission of Drug-Energy" through uprooted hair of patient has been verified in all respects. It has affected the newly born babies, persons during sleep, and animals. Subjective and objective effects have been observed. A big tumour in the neck of a dog and a cancerous growth of an orange size in the parotid gland of a patient have disappeared by Transmission. Sterility, peptic ulcer, eczema, Insomnia, neuralgia, sciatica, headache etc. have been cured. Effectiveness has been seen by my friends and disciples in innumerable cases under my guidance. Demonstrations have been given on different occasions of annual functions before the doctors, medical students and public with success. I am tempted to cite one recent case cured miraculously which could not be included in the chapter "Experimental Observations". Miss N. aged 17 of Patna had been suffering from hysteric fits daily between 5 and 6 P.M. She was diagnosed as Ignatia by me and Dr. S. nath on 1.6.70. In the night Nux Vom. 2C was transmitted from Boring Canal Road, Patna to university area, a distance of about 6 K.M. In the morning of 2.6.70 Ign. 1 M. was transmitted and she had fit at 5-50 p.m. only for 5 mmunutes instead of 15 to 30 minutes. In the morning of 3.6.70, 3/4 of solution was thrown and that much of water was added and 10 strokes were given. She had attack of fit at 6 p.m. for 2 minutes only. Again in the morning of 4.6.70 the same process was repeated and she had no attack since then. Transmission of Drug-Energy is based on the hard rock of experiences and experiments. A distance of more than 1000 K.M. from Bettiah to Jaipur. Bombay and Delhi has been covered so far. Distance is no bar. It may be transmitted to any corner of the world, and even to the moon.

It is no longer a hypothesis now. It is based on Inductive Logic where we proceed from the particular to the general. It is never a fact that I possess some spiritual power as some people remark. It can be done by any one. There is no secrecy. It is very simple and handy.

Much has been heard against this discovery of "Transmission of Drug—Energy" but praises too have been poured from different parts of the country. This is the age of scientific awakening that is why the criticism and opposition are not so vehement as it should have been before the Renaissance period. William Harvey had to face bitter criticism for his discovery of "Systematic Circulation", Vesalius, the father of modern Anatomy had been chased from Padus for revealing many anatomical truths by dissection of human body and Mechael Servetus was burnt for his discovery of the "Pulmonary Circulation". Who does not know that Christ was crucified for preaching Truth. Thanks to the scientific age ! Opposition of that degree is not being faced. People may pooh pooh in absence without cogitating on it but as soon as they see action, they keep mum atleast. Criticism is but natural when the traditional beliefs, dogmas and doctrines are hurt by any new discovery. Moreover, human mind is very very conservative and dogmatic. There are still people in the world who do not believe in Radio and Television. They think that there is some magical device. Though seeing is believing still sometimes even after personal observations and experiences people are sceptical. I have seen that even inteligentia class whose scistica and other difficult ailments have been cured by this method are sceptical to believe.

The high and only mission of the Homoeo Physician is to restore the sick to health, i.e. to cure the morbid state of health gently, rapidly and permanently. In this respect "Transmission of Drug Energy" is not lagging behind rather it has got various merits over the oral or traditional method. In every field of life, man has been making efforts to reach perfection. From bullock carts to rockets ! What a wonder ! Science today is making miracles. It has got victory over time and space. Many more are to be done which cannot be apprehended at present. Medical Science is also striving to attain perfection. No doubt, it has expanded in length and breadth but time and space have not been conquered though doctors in the foreign country can examine and control patients from a distance particularly in heart diseases. Homoeopathic Science is also trying to expand in volume but now by this discovery of "Transmission" one more dimension of height has been added.

It has conquered time and space. It proves supremacy of Homoeopathy over other 'pathies' inasmuch as no drug than the Homoeopathic is transmissible so far.

Flights of Apollos 11 and 12 were controlled from the earth without visible connection. The driver controls the vehicles by steering or a break. The players control the flight of kites in the sky, but there is no control in the field of medical therapy. Once a drug is administered there is no control over its action. In case of severe aggravation either it is antidoted or checked by other drugs to the detrimental effects on the economy. "Transmission" has supremacy over the traditional or oral method. In this case simply transmission is to be made off and aggravation is checked.

Transmission helps in selection of remedies as well as potencies. It is economic to the physician as well as to the patients. The patients have not to undergo ordeals of treatment. If one be on phone, it is easier to treat him from the doctor's chamber by taking his thorough history along with one hair from his head as being practised by me. Patient on phone rings and tell his complaints. He hold the phone and his hair is brought in contact with the selected remedy and he gets relief like magic sitting in his home. It sweeps away many drosses cropped in our practice. There are many other merits over the oral method. However, the pressing demands from different corners of the country for literature on "Transmission of Drug Energy" compelled me to write this book. I have tried my level best to give a back-ground in the first part of the book. The 2nd part deals with "Transmission" proper. misconceptions have been clarified. Human body, Nervous system, Disease, Vital force, Drug, potency and ionisation etc. have been explained.

xxxvi

Scientific explanation of Transmission and technique have been given. It has already been submitted that the potentized drug remains in the phial or globule in ionised form. It forms an electrical field in the phial. The hair has got the same characteristic vibrations as that of the body of the individual. As in the case of body, the hair also is electrically charged. When the electrical field of the drug comes in contact with that of the hair, the resultant field becomes so intense and rapid that it begins to radiate energy, waves or pulses at a particular frequency. As the Constitution and Vibratory state of the hair, which transmits the resultant energy (effect of medicine) is the same as that of the body from which the hair was detached, this vibration of hair caused by the effect of medicine causes a similar and sympathetic vibration in the body and thus the disordered economic becomes normal.

Large number of cases treated by this method, with full particulars have been given in the Chapter, "Experimental observations". Every pros and cons have been explained as far as possible.

I am conscious of limitations, omissions and commissions but I feel immense pleasures in sincere endeavor to present this book written in haste to brother Homoeopaths, scientists, doctors of other fields and those who are interested in the subject in the full hope that it will be enriched by criticisms, valuable suggestions and kind help in future. My efforts will be fruitful if this will kindle the interest and satisfy the curiosity of readers. I apologise for anything lacking or errors that may be found in the book. Suggestions and Criticisms will be cordially welcome.

B. Sahni
10.6.1970

ABOUT THE AUTHOR

Dr. Bandhu Sahni was born on 17th January, 1925 in a village called Karkouli in the district of Darbhanga. Dr. Sahni's early childhood is a tale of pain and penury. His father, being a poor cultivator, found it difficult to maintain the family with his petty income. Dr. Sahni's extraordinary intelligence and zeal for acquiring knowledge at once attracted the notice of Late Munshi Udit Narain of Rajnagar who was well-known for his love for learning and magnanimity. Under his loving care Dr. Sahni spent a couple of years at Rajnagar and passed his matriculation examination in 1942. The same year his father died, leaving him broken-hearted. However, he sought admission in I.A. classes in C.M. College, Darbhanga, but since he was a fire-brand nationalist, he could not help taking part in the freedom movement of 1942. This made him realise that no sacrifice could be considered greater than one done for the sake of one's country. It was during this period that he was attracted towards the Homoeopathic science, which to him, held promises in new awakening in poor masses. It was a chanticleer of new dawn which in its turn would bring health and happiness to the suffering humanity.

Dr. Sahni—a man of indefatigable spirit and peerless character, again in 1943 took up his studies with renewed vigour and sincerity. He graduated in 1947 from C.M. College, Darbhanga. Once he had chosen Homoeopathy as his love, he could hardly live without it and so even during his college days, he kept up his interest in it.

Dr. Sahni joined Basic Training School at Patna in 1948. He also went to Sevagram for higher training in basic education. Soon after finishing B.T. course, he was married to Dr. Sumitra Sahni, who, too, had done her basic training course from Patna Basic Training School. Both of them were appointed Assistant Teachers in Post & Senior Basic Schools at Kolhanta Patori in the district of Darbhanga respectively.

At no stage of his career, Dr. Sahni's interest in Homoeopathy flagged. While in Govt. service, he passed his M.D.

examination in Homoeopathy and got a first class. This encouraged him to establish a charitable Homoeopathic dispensary under the social education scheme. Dr. Sahni combined in him the best qualities of a doctor as well as a teacher and thus earned a good name for himself in both the fields. Dr. (Mrs.) Sahni has had a definite role to play in her husband's successful ventures. Both husband and wife were transferred to Mandar Block, Ranchi as S.E.O.S. in the beginning of 1954. They worked in this capacity for nearly four years to the entire satisfaction of all concerned. Dr. Sahni's love for learning and extraordinary zeal always helped him climb fresh heights. While in service, Dr. Sahni appeared at the M.A. Examination in Philosophy and got a high second class. The same year he competed for a gazetted post in Bihar Public Service Commission. He also took his M.A. examination in sociology and got a high second class. In his service career, Dr. Sahni had also the opportunity of successfully completing many in-service training courses organised by the Central and State Governments. While in service at Bhagalpur, Dr. Sahni came out with his research on "Transmission of Homoeopathic Drug-Energy" which was greatly appreciated by recognised centres of Homoeopathic science. In recognition of his valuable research many academic bodies and institutions for Homoeopathic science conferred upon him honorary degrees and fellowship.

While at Bettiah, (11-6-68 to 1-1-70), Dr. Sahni's health began to fail probably because of the unhealthy environment. His heart got inflicted and some trouble of gout also bothered him, which finally forced him to go on long leave from January 1, 1970. After recovery from his illness he joined as a Subdivisional Welfare Officer at Dinapur, Patna on the 15th March 1971 where he worked to the full satisfaction of the authorities. Later on promotion to a higher post he joined as a lecturer at the State Institute of Education, Bihar, Patna on 4-7-74 and has been working there since then.

Dr. Sahni has many published and unpublished papers to his credit. A great lover of books as Dr. Sahni is, he has in his library a collection of rare books on Homoeopathy. Dr. Sahni's publications, namely, (1) Transmission of Homoeo Drug-Energy From a distance." (A New Discovery) Ist Edition, (2) "Ek Dinme Doctor" (Hindi), (3) "Drug picture of Biochemistry with transmission". (4) Rog Lakshan Sangrah prapatra" (Hindi) and

(5) "Case Taking proforma with guidelines" bear testimony to his great scholarship and extraordinary insight in the field of Homoeopathic science. His wife, who is still in Govt. service, has not only been a happy partner to him, but also an active collaborator in his researches. Dr. Sahni goes on ceaselessly in search of truth and is thoroughly convinced that the gratification of self is not the only object for which one is ushered in this world. Burning self emotion is cheerless, arid and society-imposed duty. He exemplifies it in his own life. A journalist rightly called him "A Physician, a Messiah". Always anxious to think in original manner. Dr. Sahni's interpretations add di-. mension to the science of Homoeopathy.

Dr. Sahni's is the chief Editor of the chief quarterly Magazine, "HOMOEO TARNG" in Hindi.

Research Institute of Sahni Drug Transmission & Homoeopathy was established & he was made its honorary director. The Institute is registered & aid is being given by the Govt. of Bihar. The Institute has been functioning well under the able guidance of the discoverer himself. Its working and Research Methodology are attracting people all over the medicine world. This Institute has been conferring Fellowship (F.R.I.S.T.) upon the practitioners abroad & the Indian Nationals as well on completion of training and contributions.

Brajnandan Prasad

B.Sc. (Bio) B.H.U.B.S. (Fisheries) Washington
M.A.F.S., M.I.F.S.
T.I.F. (CAL.) T.F.S. (F.A.O.) Thailand
Deputy Director, Fisheries, Bihar,
PATNA

PART I

SOME RESEARCHES

CHAPTER I

SOME RESEARCHES IN HOMOEOPATHY

Introduction—After the author's discovery, "Transmission of Homoeo Drug Energy From A Distance" on the 6th January 1967, he made several experiments and wrote down an article under the caption, "Homoeo Dynamic Medicine can be Transmitted Through uprooted hair of the patient" which was published in the April 1967 issue of, "The Torch of Homoeopathy" with an encouraging editorial notes suggesting some books and articles. The author collected some more literature on researchers in the field.

A cursory glance over the history of Homoeopathy will reveal that the science of Homoeopathy is evolving like an organism from the days of Dr. S. Hahnemann. It is never static. The father of Homoeo proved a few no. of medicines but these days no. has increased and is on increase every day. A time will come when the number of medicines will increase so much that the future progeny will find difficulty in comprehending. The science is developing not only in volume but also in depth and height. Many researches and advancements have been made in the field. New approaches are being made.

Dr. Albert Abrams' works

1. The body is composed of innumerable living cells and all the cells are electrically charged. The total equilibrium is maintained by a net work of wire, i.e., nervous system, the headquarter being in the brain where news are received through the sensory nerves and orders are communicated outside through the motor nerves. Two way traffic is well maintained. The human body is emanating electromagnetic waves at the rate of 80 million cycles per second and hence it is beyond the perception of our visual capacity. Dr. Albert Abrams of San Francisco

turned his attention to the "wireless waves which emanate from the human body". While he was studying the spinal reflex of the body by percussion, he discovered the "electromagnetic waves." He found dull note of tuberculosis in almost all cases whether suffering from tuberculosis or not. He discovered that he had that dullness when the patient were facing west but he could not find that sound when the patients were turned to face north or south.

This difference is due to polarity. This fact shows the relations between the individual and the electro-magnetic field of the earth. This experiment has been verified many times.

2.   Dr. Abrams made another experiment. He held a piece of tissue containing tubercle bacilli over the neck of a healthy person and the same dull note was heard on percussion. This experiment shows that the piece of tubercular specimen emanates wireless waves which are received and recorded by the human organisms and they alter very character of the healthy tissue. From this experiment, it may be concluded that the part (or tissue) even when separated from the body emanates electromagnetic waves and influences the person brought in contact with that tissue.

3.   Another experiment of Dr. Abrams runs like this. Two persons, one suffering from T.B. and another healthy, were connected with a wire. One end of the wire was placed over the lesion on the patient and the other on the cervical vertebra of the healthy person. He obtained by tapping the back of the healthy person, the same dullness as that of the patient. That shows that the electrical waves can be transmitted from the diseased to the healthy when so connected.

4.   Now let us come to the wireless system in which without any direct connection message is received. Dr. Abrams made another discovery. He was examining a patient by percussion and he obtained a dull note on the abdomen. He could not account for that note. Then he noticed a bottle containing a cancer growth on his table. He got that bottle removed and the dull sound also disappeared. He made this experiment again and again and came to the same conclusion. This is a clear evidence of the passage of waves through space.

5.   Dr. Abrams followed another experiments with other diseases. He found that the area-reflex was not sufficient as syphilis caused a reflex on the same area as cancer. So he was

in need of a medicine to measure wave-length of disease radiations to diagnose different diseases. He got a coil wound with resistances marked in ohms. He found that the best place for the reception of the waves from the patient was the forehead of the healthy person. "He found that in case of Malaria, dullness occured with his rheostat set at 32 ohms, with tubercle at 42; with an infection due to bacillus coli at 44; with acquired syphilis at 55; with hereditary syphilis at 57; with cancer at 50; with sarcoma at 58; with a streptococcal infection at 60; and so on."

This discovery was made only for diagnostic purpose.

He used a simple apparatus for diagnosis—a round back wooden box with metallic contact points from which ran grounding wires. A short insulating wire passes from the metallic top of the box, having on its free end an aluminium electrode which is applied to the forehead of the healthy person. The working of this apparatus was as follows :— "A specimen of the patients blood was placed in the box and the experimental percussions made on the abdomen of the subject, the indicator being moved at each tapping from one ohm upwards. When a dullness of sound was perceived, the reading on the rheostat was noted. And thus, from previous experiments and readings taken from the diseased tissues, he found that the disease could be identified."

Dr. Abrams went further to experiment with drugs and was able to work out for various drugs. Quinine gave him a resistance of "32 Ohms". For sometimes he used drugs to treat the patients with the help of this apparatus but the result was not very satisfactory.

Being dissatisfied with "the opposition of disease vibrations by drug vibrations" Dr. Abrams devised another machine called Oscilloclast (wave breaker) to generate suitable vibrations to cancel the disease vibrations. But he was not so successful in treating the patients on this line though the patients were stimulated by vibrations and got some relief.

Dr. William E. Boyd & his Emanometer

On queries about the Dr. William E. Boyd's Emanometer, his son Dr. H.W. Boyd, M.B., M.R.C.P. 17 Sandyfaro Place Co. 3, states in his letter dated 5-7-65. "This is not an instrument which is on the market at all and was purely used for research purposes. It is no longer being used here".

(i)   Dr. W.E. Boyd was an eminent Physician and Scientist of Glasgow. He was born in 1884 and died in 1954. He, many years after patient research showed the body-mind inter-relationship by cathoderay Oscillograph. According to him electrical activity of the body can be shown in various ways by biophysical methods.

(ii) "The skin carries varying electrical potentials which can be measured."

(iii) "There is electrical field surrounding the body extending in every direction."

(iv) "The brain activity is accompanied by electric potentials detected by modern methods of encephalography."

(v)   "The body continuously emits radiation in the long infrared regions which can be filtered by various crystals and detected by delicate thermo-junctions".

"All these activities and properties are based on electronic or atomic changes."

"The lower attenuations of Homoeo drugs, called low potencies can be shown to have their definite electro-physical properties", for example :—

(i)   "Arsenic in an attenuation of 1×10^{-7} is capable of showing distinctive response to ultra violet radiation by florescence."

(ii) "Tincture of gold prepared by the method laid down by Hahnemann, an apparently clear transparent fluid, can be shown by spectroscope methods to be capable of modifying a beam of ultra-violet light. The modification is distinctive for gold. This tincture is an attenuation of 1 in 10^{-7} i.e. 1 part in 10,000,000.

(iii) "China, the famous Cinchona of Hahnemann's early experiments, can be shown capable of physical action in ultraviolet light (Selective absorption) in an attenuation of 1×10^{-7}."

(iv) "Nux Vomica can be shown to have a similar action in an attenuation 1×10^{-5}".

(v)   "Radium bromide can by Geiger Caunter be shown to have a radiation through air (showing ionising properties) which can ultimately be visually recorded by Oscillograph in an attenuation of 1×10^{-7} and can be demonstrated by electroscope at least to 1×10^{-10} or 1 part in 10,000,000,000." (Some recent research and advancement in Homoeopathy compiled by Dr. P. Sankaran, L.I.M.D., F.H.M. (Lond) Page 1-3).

"Dr. Boyd modified and improved Dr. Abrams' box and constructed an accurate apparatus called Emanometer to detect the disease emanations and the corresponding drug radiations. A drop of some secretion of the patient as for example Salivary etc. is put on a sterile blotting paper and it is placed in one compartment of the Emanometer. A healthy subject is made to stand naked inside a screening cage in the machine and he is exposed to radiation from this secretion. The subject is well screened so that external electro-physico energies may not stand in the way. The operator thrusts his arm through a panel for percussing and two copper cloth sleeves fit in closely over his wrists. The subject is exposed to the secretion of the patient and all the while his abdomen is percussed continuously."

"When a change in the percussion note on the abdomen is noticed, the distance at which such change is produced is noted and on the basis of this the patient is assigned to a particular Emanometer Group. Then those drugs from this group are selected which seem likely to cover the symptomatology of the case and the potencies of these drugs are placed in the apparatus so that the subject is exposed simultaneously both to the disease energy and drugs energy. When the change in the percussion note caused by exposure to the patient's secretion is neutralised completely by simultaneous exposure to a drug in potency, then this drug is found to be the similimum."

Dr. Boyd had to face a highly critical committee under Chairmanship of Sri Thomas Horder and was satisfied with the results of Emanometer though the Committee was critical of the claims of Abrams' Apparatus. A series of tests were arranged to find out if potency could be identified by Bio-physical method. Dr. Boyd was able to demonstrate to differentiate between the various potencies of Sodium Chloride such as 30,200 and 100000. Not only that, the Emanometer was able to distinguish between various drugs like Arsenic, Pulsatilla, Belladona, Calcium Carbonate etc. in high potencies. The Committee was satisfied with the Emanometer which could be able to detect the activity of Homoeo potencies though the chemical analysis of the potencies could not find out the medicine. Dr. Boyd proved that energies of a very delicate nature are inherent in highly potentised drugs which can evoke reactions in human organs.

Dr. P.Sankaran, L.I.M., D.F. Hom. (Lond) Hon. Physician, Government Homoeopathic Hospital, Bombay points out in "Some Recent Research and Advances in Homoeopathy" that similar but simple experiment can be carried out by any one. This experiment was carried out by the author and found it to be true.

A normal person aged 17, was made to stand facing east, percussion was made over his chest at the border of the heart, one man was asked to come slowly towards the subject with an open vial containing sulphur 200 in liquid. The percussion note was changed, when he was approaching the subject at the distance of twelve meters.

The effects by the radiations from the drugs are not only confined to percussion notes but the radiation of drugs is influencing all those who handle the potentised drugs. It is being experienced in daily practice. Sometimes the effects are felt in head, in eyes and in other parts of the body. Once Dr. N.K.P. Sinha Munsif got a severe effect and he fell down with violent headache by radiation of Aconite 30 which was transmitted by him to a baby suffering from fever. Then Nux Vom. 30 was transmitted by the author to neutralise its action and his headache vanished like magic.

The Pulse Test

"The pulse test is performed as follows:—First of all twelve vials called Group vials, each containing Homoeopathic potencies, are prepared. Each group vial represents one group of Emanometer classification of drugs and is composed of a number of representative drugs drawn from the list of drugs in the Emanometer group and mixed together. For example, group vial is made up by mixing up a number of drugs of the same potency, i.e. 200 c from Emanometer group 7. Then these vials are placed on a table about two feet away from the patient. The patient is seated comfortably and his pulse is felt till it shows a steadiness in rate and rhythm. Its rate is then noted by counting for two or three minutes. Now the group vials containing the potencies are brought either very close to the patient or into contact with his arm quickly one by one in succession. Even if the vials are corked the potencies influence the patient, while the vial is in contact with the patient. The pulse rate is counted for 15 seconds. Then this vial is put away and the next group vial is taken up. It is best before testing the next vial to "sort" the patient by asking him to hold a metal bar with both hands so that a circuit is formed from one side of his body to the other. As each group vial is tested, a note is made as to which group vial tends to normalise the pulse most; slowing it if it is fast, accelerating it if it is slow."

"Now from among the remedies in this particular group these drugs are selected which appear to cover the symptomatology of the case in the same way as the group vials were tested. If several drugs produce an effect the first time they are tested again and again until by a process of elimination one drug is arrived at which clearly produces the greatest normalisation of the pulse. This best single drug may sometimes alter the pulse rate by 8 or 10 beats a minute. A difference of atleast 4 beats is necessary to indicate a good remedy."

"The changes in the pulse as well as in the other reflexes observed, no doubt, result from the interaction of the disease and drug energies, this interaction being expressed through the automatic nervous system of the body. It may be said that so far these are probably the only method by which the drug energy and disease energy are detectable and measurable."

The Emanometer being a complex apparatus could not be made popular as it appears from the very pen of his son. The pulse test seems to be cumbersome. No doubt these researches in Homoeopathy open a new era though it is merely for diagnostic purpose. Testing various drugs as in the above methods & devices, on the healthy subjects or on the sick may produce drug diseases & make the cases complicated. Every drug right or wrong produces some effects on the subjects or those who handle drugs. Sometimes the results are violent as in case of Dr. Sinha but generally the actions are mild. This is the reason why these scientists used to perform experiments with a number of drugs without facing much difficulty, but this practice never rules out the possibility of violent reactions if there be any, as already discussed above.

CHAPTER II

MEDICAL RADIESTHESIA

Every thing of the universe—animate or inanimate has its own individuality, its own peculiarity and stands in relation to each other, one influences the other. Two-way traffic is seen everywhere. It gives and takes. Matter is energy and energy is matter. Dr. Albert Abrams established the doctrine known as "Electron Theory of Matter" from which has evolved the "Atomic Theory" of today. In the previous chapter it has been submitted how Dr. Abrams introduced a celebrated device to detect the disease radiations of the human body. Every object has its own reaction. These reactions spread in the world through radiations. "Every living or non-living thing attracts these radiations and either earths it or disperses it." All living matter gives off radiations. The human bodies are radio-active in this sense.

They emit or receive these radiations. Radiesthesia is an instrument or device which is based on these radiations. It detects the radiation given off by human organism and finds out the diseased organ and helps the ailing beings.

Dr. John A. Hobbs says in his article published in the "Torch of Homoeopathy" Jaipur, Rajsthan October, 1961 issue on page 236 under the head "Radiesthesia or Radionic Diagnosis" that Radiesthesia is the detection by human sensitivity of ultra fine radiations which are given off by all "living matter. Our own bodies are themselves radioactive. This is because all body cells contain potassium and all samples of potassium contain a trace of its radioactive isotope K 40".

"There is a great variation in the sensitivity of people, in both emitting and receiving these radiations. Radiesthesia is the science which deals with the determination of disease by methods which rely on the radionic response of living tissue, be it in health or disease. This method is being used by a certain number of medical men, particularly in England and the continent. It is a most exacting and arduous method, but it gives results which no other method can give, as it covers the whole subject of human radiations. There are various ways in which these sensitive radiations can be detected, perhaps the most usual being the pendulum, either on its own or used in conjunction with various types of amplifying instruments. I have been a user of a pendulum for a number of years before purchasing a Delawarr Diagnostic Machine from the Delawarr Laboratories of Oxford, England, approximately four years ago. Since then I have examined some 450 to 500 blood spots and have been amazed with the results found, as have also my patients".

"Roughly the procedure is for a small smear of blood or urine to be taken from a patient on a special clean paper. This is placed in a special receptacle in the Delawarr machine and the machine turned into the pain conditions reposted, as in turning a wireless set to a certain station. This gives a basis to commence with then tune into the rate for various organs of the body, thus ascertain which of these are affected. This sometimes entails quite a lot of cross checking, and finally we are able to find out the physical vitality rate of that organ. By so eliminating the various organs affected we find the worse one and so are able to treat that one first. Quite often it is one which whilst being the cause of most of the trouble does not indicate (itself) to the patient himself or herself much bother, i.e. pain or discomfort. Thus by the slow elimination of the various parts of the body we are able to remove not only the effect but the cause of the trouble, which is of course more important. We are able also to find out to recommend the necessary food, Homoeopathic chemical or vitamins as well as electrical or other treatment needed to assist in the correction of the condition".

Andre Simoneton, a French engineer designed a device for selection of suitable and healthy food for people. It is a simple pendulum attached to a short piece of string used by divers of water, lost object, or the future.

The art of dowsing is very ancient and has been practised since long by Chinese, Hindus, Egyptians, Persians, Greek and Romans. In the Renaissance it was revived by Christopher Von Schenberg, the director of Mines in Saxony.

In the Soviet Union geologists have recently been "dowsing for minerals from airplanes and also locating underground archaeological artifacts". "The mecca for dowsers in Europe is located in a small Parisian side street, now lost between the luxury of the Faubourg Saint Honore and the tourist-ridden arcades of the rue de Rivoli, appropriately named for Saint Roch, Canonized for protecting the populace against various pestilences. The actual Kaaba is an old Curiosity shop called the Maison de Radiesthesie, "Radiesthesie' being generic for dowsing and for the search for *radiations beyond the electromagnetic spectrum*, an appellative given to the art by the Abbe Bouly, who coined it from the Greek for "Sensitivity" and the Latin for "radiance". "In the scientific community the art is now on the fringe of recognition".

The specific technique of dowsing food for freshness and vitality was learned by engineer, Simoneton from Andre Bovis. According to the Bovis' theory the "earth has positive magnetic currents running north to south, negative magnetic currents running east to west. He says that these currents are picked up by all bodies on the surface of the earth, and that any body placed in a north-south position will be more or less polarized, depending on its shape and consistency. In human bodies these telluric currents, both positive and negative, enter through one leg and go out through the opposite hand. At the same time cosmic currents from beyond the earth enter through the head and go out through the other hand and foot. The currents also go out through the open eyes".

"All bodies containing water, says Bovis, accumulate these currents and can radiate them slowly. As the currents go out and act and react against other magnetic forces in objects, they affect the pendulum held by the dowser. Thus human bodies, as a variable condenser, acts as a detector, selector and amplifier of short and ultra-short waves; it is a go-between for the animal electricity of Galvani and the inanimate electricity of Volta".

"At the same time the pendulum says Bovis, acts as a perfect lie detector in that if a person is frankly saying what he thinks about some subject, it will not affect the radiations and thus not affect the pendulum; but anyone saying something different from what he is thinking changes the wave lengths, making them shorter and negative".

Bovis developed a pendulum from crystal with a fixed metal point suspended on a double strand of red and violet silk. He called it "Paradiamagnetique" because it is sensitive to objects which are either attracted or repelled by a magnet. Bodies, which are attracted, such as iron, cobalt, magnesium etc. are called by him, "Paramagnetic" and those which are repelled, such as copper, zinc, tin, lead, sulfur and bismuth are called, "diamagnetic". By placing a small magnetic field in the form of a solenoid between the dowser and the pendulum, he claimed to be able to pick up very faint currents such as those emanating from a nonfecundated egg. He explained the use of red and violet strands as increasing the sensitivity of his pendulum on the grounds that red light vibrations are the same as the atomic vibrations of iron, which are paramagnetic and those violet being the same as Copper which are diagmagnetic.

Bovis claimed that he could tell the intrinsic vitality and relative freshness of different foods due to their power of radiations and also measure with his pendulum, their varying radiant frequencies. For this purpose Bovis developed a 'BIOMETRE' arbitrarily graduated in centimeters to indicate microns, which are thousandths of a millimeter, and angstroms, which are a hundred times smaller, covering a band between zero and ten thousand angstroms. By placing a piece of fruit or vegetable, or any kind of food he could measure its vitality with the help of the Biometre.

"Simoneton found that food which radiates 8,000 to 10,000 angstroms on Bovis' Biometre' would also cause a pendulum to Turn at the remarkable speed of 400 to 500 revolutions per minute in a radius of 80 millimeters. Foods which radiate between 6,000 and 88,000 spun it at a rate of 300 to 400, with a radius of 60 millimeters. Meats, pasteurized milk, and overcooked vegetables, which radiate less than 2,000 angstroms, have not sufficient energy to make the pendulum spin."

"For those who might complain about the arbitrary selection of angstroms for measuring the relative radiant vitality of objects, Louis Kervran, in a preface to Simoneton's book, *Radiations des Aliments*, points out that the angstrom is no more arbitrary than the calorie used in nutrition, a calorie being the quantity of heat required to raise the temperature of one gram of water one degree centigrade. All systems of measurement, says Kervran, are conventional; Bovis' angstrom merely made it easy to distinguish between the radiant value of fermented cheese, which reads at 1,500 and that of fresh olive oil, which reads at 8,5000. In any case Kervran adds, the wave lengths emitted by fruits and vegetables and other biochemical food stuffs which are picked up with the pendulum are of totally unknown nature, apparently outside the electromagnetic spectrum. It is simply the fact that they are measurable by dowsing methods which remain of great practical value".

"According to Bovis, wave lengths broadcast by an object are picked up by the nerves in a human arm and then amplified by means of a pendulum swinging at the end of a string. Impressive proof of this has been established in Montreal by Jan Jerat, whose laboratory experiments clearly indicate that a minute muscular movement occurs in the area of the wrist second after a change in the encephalograph has been registered. Merta has also designed a dowsing device, which can be placed not only in the hands but on the arms, shoulders, head, legs, or feet, or any other part of the body where it can be balanced".

"In line with Bovis and Lakhovsky, Simoneton reasoned that if human nerve cells can receive wave lengths they must also be transmitters; senders and receivers must be able to enter into resonant vibration with each other in order to pick up a transmission. Lakhovsky likened the system to two well tuned pianos : when a note is struck on one it will cause the same note to vibrate on the other".

"Dehydrated fruit was found by experiment to retain its vitality; if soaked in "vitalized" water for twenty-four hours, even several months after drying, it would radiate almost as strongly as when freshly picked. Canned fruits remained perfectly dead. Water turned out to be a very strange medium : normally unradiant, it was capable of being "vitalized" by association with minerals, human beings, or plants. Some waters, such as those at Lourdes, Bovis found, in 1926, to radiate as high as 156,000 angstroms. Eight years later some of the same water still registered 78,000 angstroms. The Czech-born psychic Jan Merta holds that the rind from apples, pears, and other fruits and vegetables, when left to soak in a glass of water overnight, releases healthful vibrations into the water which can then be drunk to provide better nourishment than the rind itself, which has little or no effect on Simoneton's pendulum".

Simoneton says fruits are filled with solar radiation in the healthful light spectrum between the bands of infrared and ultra violet, and that their radiance rises slowly to a peak while ripening, then gradually decreases to zero at putrefaction. The banana, which is healthily edible for about eight days out of a span of twenty-four between the time it is picked and when it starts to rot, gives off optimum vibrations when it is yellow, not so good when green, and very low when black".

"Vegetables are most radiant if eaten raw, two raw carrots being better than a plateful of cooked ones. The potato, which has a radiance of only 2,000 angstroms when raw (perhaps because it grows underground hidden from the sun), mysteriously rises to 7,000 angstroms when boiled and all the way to a very healthy 9,000 when baked. The same applies to other tubers".

"Legumes, such as peas, beans, or chickpeas, rate 7,000 to 8,000 fresh. Dried they lose most of their radiance. They become heavy, indigestible, and hard on the liver, says Simoneton. To benefit from legumes they too should be eaten raw and freshly picked. Optimum results, says Simoneton, come from their juices, especially if drunk at 10 A.M. and 5 P.M. when they are easily digested and do not tire the system but nourish it".

"On Simoneton's scale wheat has a radiance of 8,500 angstroms; when cooked this rises to 9,000. He says wheat can and should be eaten in a variety of ways rather than simply in bread. Whole wheat flour should mixed into pies, tarts, and other pastries with butter, eggs, milk, fruits, and vegetables. Baked in a wood burning oven, bread gives off even better radiations than if cooked with coal or gas".

"Olive oil was found by Simoneton to have a high radiance of 8,500, and to be extremely long-lasting. Six years after pressing it still gives off around 7,500. Butter, which radiates about 8,000, is good for about ten days before it starts to fall off, reaching bottom in about twenty days".

"Ocean fish and shell fish are good foods with a bright radiance from 8,500 to 9,000 especially if caught fresh and eaten raw. This includes crabs, oysters, clams, and other shell fish. Lobsters, says Simoneton, are best cut in half while live and boiled on a wood fire. Fresh water fish is much less radiant".

"In Simoneton's second category he places foods radiating from 6,500 down to 3,000 angstroms. These include eggs, peanut oil, wine, boiled vegetables, cane sugar, and cooked fish. He rates a good red wine between 4,000 and 5,000, and says it is a better drink than devitalized city water, and certainly better

than coffee, chocolate, liquor, or pasteurized fruit juices, which
have virtually no radiance".

"Echoing Nichols, Simoneton says that, whereas the juice
of a fresh sugar beet gives 8,500 angstroms, refined beet sugar
can fall as low as 1,000, and the white lumps that get wrapped
in papers are down to zero".

"Of meats, the only one that makes Simoneton's list of
edible foods is freshly smoked ham. Freshly killed pork radiates
at 6,500, as does all animal meat; but once it has been soaked in
salt and hung over a wood fire its radiance rises to 9,500 or
10,000 angstroms. Other meats are almost pointless to eat; they
are an exercise in tough digestion, which wars out rather than
vitalizes the eater, requiring him to drink coffee to keep from
falling asleep".

"Cooked meats, sausages, and other innards are all in
Simoneton's third category along with coffee, tea, chocolate,
jams, fermented cheeses, and white bread. Because of their low
radiation they do one little or no good, says Simoneton".

"In his fourth category are margarines, preserves, alco-
hols, liquors, refined white sugar, and bleached white flour : all
dead as far as radiations are concerned".

"Applying his technique for measuring wave lengths
directly to human beings, Simoneton found that the normal
healthy person gives off a radiance of about 6,500 or a little
higher, whereas the radiations given off by tobacco smokers,
alcohol imbibers, and carrion eaters are uniformly lower. Bovis
claimed that cancer patients give off a wave length of 4,875,
which, he noted, was the same wave length as that of over
refined white French bread before the Second World War".

"It struck Simoneton that the therapeutic marvels attributed since the dawn of history to herbs, flowers, roots, and barks
might not be due simply to their chemical content, but the
healthy wave lengths they radiate. Though the apothecary's
shelves are still stocked with chemical derivatives from plants
and herbs, their curative powers no longer appear so miraculous. The secret of their potency seems to have been lost".

"Useful as it is to use Radiesthesia as an adjunct to
pathological diagnosis, it is time it was used in its proper
sphere—the sphere of health and wholeness, when it can measure the degree of the whole body, where one thinks in terms of

whole body health, and not in just the effect of a part in pain. Now-a-days it would appear, that man is no longer considered as a whole, but treated according to the individual whim of the person handling the case," Radiesthesia is also being used in our country by Dr. T. Sinha, 271, Tula Ram Bagh, Allahabad and others. Dr. Sinha has got rich experiences in this field. He is the author of "Medical Rediesthesia" written in simple and clear language. In his book he has given a historical sketch of Radiesthesia. It was in use in 2000 B.C. but gradually it faded with the advent of materialism.

Radiesthesia is based on the radiation of cosmic rays. "Various kinds of electric currents pass in the atmosphere. Some of them are natural while others are artificial. The natural electric currents which move by radiation have mostly the magnetic origin, like the rays of sun which taking the form of electric waves get radio-active. The artificial current of waves are those which are broadcasted by man made instruments. Every electric current which moves by radiation seeks earth through a good conductor from the atmosphere. Every living organism of this world is a good conductor and so becomes a good medium for earthing these currents. On this supposition as its basis the Radiesthesia has been evolved".

"According to the principles of magnetism and electricity, the radiation of any energy is influenced by every object, whether a good or a bad conductor. If any good conductor comes in their path, these currents pass through that good conductor at a rapid speed and velocity, get embedded in the earth. In the case of a bad conductor the currents move away from it, such conductors, obstruct it. Every object has its own individual capacity. The desire to discover some device to detect these radiations and put them to some use, is the motive which has brought Radiesthesia to light".

Instead of instrument "Oscilloclast" of Dr. Abrams, the pendulum is used. It is made of metal as well as of wood. Dr. Sinha on his experience advocates the wooden pendulum which is the best according to him. The pendulum can be prepared anywhere. It can be made of Sheesham wood of shape and size of duck egg. Its broader end should be pierced to make a hole through which a silken cord of 15 inches may be passed. A cotton reel also may be used as pendulum.

Methods of Experiments and Its Applications

Every experiment needs equipments suited to its method-ology. Radiesthesia should have following requisites to achieve its end :—

1. A suitable place with fresh air and proper light away from noises etc. The room should be furnished with as less number of good conductors as possible or they will disturb the experiment.

2. Time—it should be in the morning say between 4 and 10 A.M.

3. The experimenter should have patience and mental equi-librium otherwise the result will not be satisfactory.

4. A pendulum—the knobs of the pendulum should be wooden-abony.

5. Charts.

6. Medicines.

7. Patient or sample of the patient in forms of blood or any of his belongings.

"At appropriate time and proper environment and at the convenient place, the experimenter should sit on a wooden chair, with wooden table close in front of him, away from the walls, facing west, with the pendulum. He should put down his bare feet on the ground firmly in such a manner that his left hand on the table is in a position that his fingers should be pointing towards the sample. Holding the silk cord between his little finger and the thumb of his right hand, he should observe the motion of the pendulum". When the pendulum comes over the sample, only the following position would be noticed. These indicate different results :—

   (i) Pendulum may become motionless and become still. It indicates that the experimenter should put off his experiment.

   (ii) The motion of the pendulum may be in a straight line. This points to the conclusion that the sample pos-sesses in plenty magnetic power and like a magnet it has acquired 'poles'. Besides this, the particular motion shows that the sample is useless for our purpose and with it we are not likely to acquire success.

(iii) The pendulum may acquire circular motion. This motion can be clockwise or anti-clockwise. Clockwise motion is positive while anti-clockwise is negative.

(iv) "Mixed motion of the pendulum is the fourth position. This proves that the mental state of the experimenter is not conducive and he should postpone his attempts till his mind gets composed".

The pendulum is suspended at least two inches above the surface of the table.

The experimenter should take his seat and make the patient sit on a chair before him. Then the patient should rotate it pausing at each region of the inner side of the left hand palm. The negative rotation of the pendulum from his right hand should be noted and the particular organ to be found out. This, it would become known which organ in particular is affected and is performing disfunction. During the experiment, experimenter and the patient should take all the things off.

The Method of Selection of Medicine

"The selection of medicine is possible with the co-operation of the patient in his presence and even in his absence. The experimenter should seat the patient facing him, then with his left hand he should hold the right hand of the patient. He should get all the probable remedies arranged in a circle on the table. A piece of white paper must be placed on which the remedy should be kept, this is to prevent any possible error. The pendulum should then be allowed to oscillate over the remedy. One, over which, it moves in a clockwise direction, is the indicated remedy. Though it seems so simple to describe, it is very difficult in practice and takes a lot of time".

Medicine may be selected even in absence of the patient. In this case his sample in the form of his blood is used. Blood is taken on a blotting paper. This blotting paper is placed on the table on a piece of white paper. The probable remedies are arranged in a circle on the table with slips of white paper beneath each remedy. The pendulum is suspended on each remedy, the one over which it oscillates in a clockwise direction is the indicated remedy.

Dr. T. Sinha, opines that by various methods potency of the medicine can also be found out. Though this method cannot fully discover the potency homoeopathically. Yet the nearest to the standard scale of medicinal potency can be reached. The method for finding out this is the same which is used in the selection of a remedy. Dr. Sinha has a better percentage of success in experiments done with samples than in the presence of the patient.

From the above submissions the readers will see that any belonging to the patient represents his individuality. Even his shirts, coat etc. may used as samples. His blood or his dress recently put off emanates electric current for the use of Radiesthesia. It influences the pendulum from a distance, i.e. the electric current emanated from the sample is transmitted to the pendulum and it oscillates to indicate the right remedy or potency.

From the use of Radiesthesia it can be safely concluded that electric current is transmitted from the sample or the patient to the pendulum from a distance.

Dr. Chandra Prakash in his editorial note on Dynamic Actions of Drugs & Plants by their external exhibition from distance by Dr. B.N. Saxena, in the "Torch of Homoeopathy" quotes from "An Introduction to Medical Radiesthesia and Radionics".

"Dr. Ruth Drown in the U.S. and the Delawarr Laboratories in England, have carried out work of major importance in designing compact radionic instruments for diagnosis and for broadest treatment, whereby an instrument is tuned to the blood-spot of the patient and specific radiations thought by some to be of electro-magnetic type are broadcasted through the ether to the patient, wherever he may be".

It is suggested that any one who has never handled the pendulum before, may try as a first experiment with a cotton reel. A cotton reel may be suspended by a fine thread of 4½ to 6 inches. The cotton reel may be suspended over various articles of food. It is better to place such article in turn on a clean sheet of white paper. It will be found that the pendulum will move in a clockwise direction if the food is suitable to the person concerned, in an anti-clockwise direction if it is unsuitable, while if it is neither good or bad, the pendulum will oscillate in a straight line. This can be done.

CHAPTER III

ACUPUNCTURE,
ZONE THERAPY AND YOGA

The human organism is a self-repairing and self-healing system. Dr. F.K. Bellokossy says in his article, "There is no medicine" that the man does not need any medicine, rather medicine has no existence. There are only two things—poison and food. He needs food. It is useless to think that the physician will repair the diseased cells of the body in the same way as the mechanics repair the motor car. He can only help the cells by supplying proper food. The non-eatable is foreign to the cells and they have to fight it out hence when administered, it is rejected by the organism. His statement is supported by various methods of treatments. In China there is no word (terminology) for medicine. There is one symbol which indicates medicine as well as poison. There is a 3000 years old method of treatment called "ACUPUNCTURE" in which no medicine is needed for any disease. All diseases are claimed to be cured by this primitive system.

This system originated in China but gradually with introduction of the modern system of treatment it began to decline in its mother land and took shelter in Japan. Even after introduction of modern system in Japan people did not leave it. It was taken up in the right earnest. Researches were done & improvement was made in Acupuncture. There are many doctors practising this system. From Japan it spread to the western countries but it was not cordially welcome due to the very idea of prick. It gives an unpleasant feeling to the patients. Some physicians are practising it in France and in India.

Acupuncture means a prick of a needle. The acupuncturists introduce very fine needles into the skin on the specific points according to diseases. 14 "meridians" and 800 points have been discovered in the body so far. The acupuncturists talk of "Ch'." the "vital energy" or "life force". According to the theory of acupuncture energy flows along "meridians" connecting the

"acupoints" on the surface of the body. According to the Chinese
the vital energy is polarized into the positive & negative "Yang"
& "Yin". There is a constant interplay of the mind & the body,
and the environment. These are linked with the vital energy.
This energy is constantly fluctuating due to changes in seasons,
weather, climate, illness, emotions, tension, thoughts etc. The
highest healing Science works with the invisible "Ch'i" energy
and the pricks of needles balance in energy is maintained. Every
individual is unique hence he needs individual treatment. No
two patients are alike "Each must be viewed as a whole by the
vital energy in a unique relationship with the whole creation".

According to the Chinese philosophy there are two realities (dualism) "Yang & Yin". The man is healthy if equilibrium
is maintained by the balance of Yang & Yin. Yang is the external
energy and Yin is internal. The former indicates sun, light, heat,
brilliance etc. While Yin indicates night, cold, darkness etc. The
first is life while the second is cause of death. One comes from
heaven while the other comes from within. They are dynamic
forces. According to the Chinese both are flowing incessantly. If
needle is pricked at a particular acupoint, there is a wave of
peculiar sensation and it seems that some thing is entering the
body along a line and that "something" is Chinese "Tsri". Yang
is pure essence while the yin is pure material. This philosophy
resembles sankhya system of India.

"All the principles of nature are derived from one basic
law, the oscillation of yin & yang. The mutations of yin & yang
represent the universal force of Tao. In the Tao, yin is receptive
and Yang is active. Their function is mutation & the result of
their interaction is continual creation. In every element of life
there is both yin & yang. In one is contained the seed of the
other. In life is the seed of death. In death is the seed of life."

Acupuncture treats illness of the body's organs by recre-
ating a proper equilibrium. It brings yin & yang into balance
and good health results.

There are 12 bilateral symmetric meridians which are
connected with each other. Besides these there are two medi-
cines-one outer and another inner. They are meant for particular organs with different functions. 10 meridians meant for
heart, stomach, liver, colon, intestine, lungs, pancreas, kidney,
urinary bladder & gall bladder.

Another allied method of oriental treatment is massage

and China is its birth place also. It is also a very old practice. It is considered as the most natural and restorative technique. To understand its technique & idea it is essential to know the dualistic monism of China which has already been described partially.

The Taoist philosopher has written that one produces two, two produces three and three is manifested in all possible beings. Commenting on the cosmology of yin and yang Ohsawa says "one produces two. . . . we understand by two, the two activities yin and yang; this is the polarization of their universe. These two give rise to all living and inert things. In this statement, one sees set forth the theory of polarized monism, and the theory of the evolution of the universe and all creation. The yin & yang theory is not ordinary dualism because there is no being, nor any phenomenon purely yin or purely yang; all are extremely varied manifestations of the possible combinations of the two activities."

This is the natural process of Tao, the order of the universe, all pervasive flow of existence. "Therefore, in massage the practitioner attempts to create an energy circuit with his patient by developing a polarity of electromagnetic charge between himself and his patient. This polarity is never expressed as a purely intellectual concept, but as an actual physician relationship and entails a passage of "vital energy" "life essence" "Ch'i" or "Ki" as it is called, between the practitioner and patient. The practitioner must be stronger than his patient"—The equilibrium of the Ki of the patient is maintained by the massage techniques similar to the techniques in acupuncture. The massage tries to "Stimulate" or "Charge" the Ki of the patient by channelising his own Ki. In massage the patient as whole is treated and not his particular organ.

There is great similarity between massage or acupuncture and Homoeopathy. Dr. S. Hahnemann himself has recommended massage along with the Homoeopathic treatment. In Homoeopathy the vital principle is stimulated by introduction of subtle energy of potentised drug and by massage or acupuncture vital energy is introduced into the body. Due to this similarity acupuncture has been introduced in the syllabus of the Homoeopathic college in France. Both systems work with small stimuli. Massage or acupuncture and Homoeopathy treat the patient as a whole and not a disease. Both are harmless and

quite in accordance with the process of nature. Both deal with
vital energy "Ki" in massage or acupuncture & vital principle in
Homoeopathy.

From the above lines it would be clear now that energy is
introduced into the body through acupoints along meridians or
nervous system from outside and equilibrium of vital energy of
the human organism is maintained without any medicine. This
method of introducing energy may be called a direct method due
to direct connection between needles & the body.

This method of treatment (Acupuncture) creats terror &
unpleasant feeling in the patients. It seems cruel & cumbersome.

Zone Therapy :

The Zone therapy reminds the author of his past experiences. In case of colic he used to bind his legs just above the
ankles tightly with clothes and in a few minutes he was free
from troubles. It was experimented on many patients also. In
case of headache he used to bind his left arm tightly with cloth
and after a few minutes his left hand was numb resulting in
complete recovery. There is a practice of using a pair of wooden
sandles each comprising of the bottom on which rests the foot
with a small vertical post with a neck around which the big toe
and the next toe rest and thus enabling the wearer to have a grip
on it. When a person walks wearing them, nerves between toes
are pressed. It is said that this practice controls the sexual
excitement and hydroceles, and hence it is generally practised
by the sages and saints. Parasu Ram & Narada, the Indian seers
of the religious scriptures have been depicted wearing these
wooden sandles. These practices are probably based on the zone
therapy.

However, the Zone therapy is a system discovered many
years ago by William H. FitzGerald M.D. of Hartford, Conn. Dr.
Fitz Geral is a graduate of the Vermont University & he spent
two & one half years in the Boston city Hospital. This therapy
is known more widely throughout the U.S.A. "The modern
theory of zone therapy is that crystaline deposits form at the
nerve endings. These keep the electrical contact or impulse of
the nerves from grounding". In zone therapy these crystaline
deposits are rubbed out to enable the nerves to ground in the
feet, hands or wherever it is chosen to work.

"In zone therapy the body is divided longitudinally into
ten zones, five on each side of a median line". The first, second,

third, fourth & fifth zone begin in the toes and end in the thumbs and fingers. The first zone extends from the great toe up the entire height of the body from infront to back, across the chest & the back & down the arm into the thumb or vice-versa".

The tongue is also divided into ten longitudinal zones, five on each side of the median line. In the same way the hard and soft palate have been divided into ten longitudinal zones, five on each side of the median line.

"Pain in any part of the first zone may be treated and overcome by pressure on all surfaces of the joint of the great toe or the corresponding joint of the thumb. Firm pressure on the end of the great toe or tip or thumb controls the entire first zone and pressure on tips of the fingers controls the individual zones.

In this way ailments are controlled by firm pressure on specified zones. Certain instruments are also used to press the particular zones. Aluminium combs, rubber bands, palate-pressor electrode, clamps, eye-muscle retractor, nasal probe, tongue pressor electrode, stickpins, lighted match etc. are used for treatment different ailments of the body.

General pain, headache, goitre, deafness, nervous tension, lumbago, fever, asthma Tonsillitis, Whooping coughs, tumor, troubles of teeth, Arthritis etc. have been cured successfully by the zone therapy.

Zone therapy can save thousands of lives if learnt & practised properly. It is worth learning & every family must know this art. It may save much if taken up properly. People consume drugs for pains and have to suffer their side-effects. By practice of this therapy one may save himself from ill-effects of overdrugging.

Yoga:

The Yoga philosophy is the priceless gift of the great Indian sage. It was evolved from the Vedas, the most ancient scriptures of India. "It is as ancient as India herself and as modern as the space age." It lays down a practical path for attaining liberation. It is the law of life. It means union of human consciousness with the universal consciousness. It also means rediscovery of the bliss in man, which he has lost due to lack of introvertion, self-enquiry and inner and outer purity. The aim of Yogic practices is to achieve the peace, power and spiritual wisdom as well as perfect health, sound mind & balanced personality. It cures many physical, mental and psychic diseases and abnormalities. It arouses all the latent potentialities of man. It gives a spiritual realization & destroys all kinds of ignorance and thus establishes brotherhood & unity between man & man. Yoga means the science of deep and subtle phenomenon of human awareness and organic functions. It "embodied" the secrets of successful living and combines profound & age-old truths with a way of acceptable to the modern mind.

The Yogic practices help man in getting rid of impurities and lead him to higher goal. "The basic principles of purification underlines all Yogic practices and at the same time it aims at establishing a balance in the body so that it functions as it were, like a perfect machine. When this state of physical balance is achieved the mind can then be controlled & he can realize the ultimate in pure thought & reason". It "aims at harmony and equilibrium of the potentialities and aspects of human beings whether emotions, intellect, intuition etc. so that the individual can obtain the fullest possible expression of himself. Once this is obtained, then true contentment arises, until this total expression and development of personality is achieved, man will remain unhappy."

There are three paths of Yoga:—Jnana (knowledge) Bhakti (Devotion) and Karma (action), each of which may lead to goal i.e. liberation.

The Yoga gives us eight fold means for purification and enlightenment of Chitta or the mind to achieve that goal. They are the disciplines of (1) Yama or restraint, (2) Niyam or culture, (3) Asana or posture, (4) Pranayama or Breath control, (5) Pratyahara or withdrawal of the senses, (6) Dharna or attention, (7) Dhyana or meditation and (8) Samadhi or concentration. They are aids to Yoga. The first three are essential for maintenance of good health. For the purpose of treatment Asana and pranayama are to be practised. Asana is a discipline of the body and consists in the adoption of steady and comfortable postures. There are various kind of Asanas such as padmasána, (Lotus pose) Virasana, (Hero pose) Bhadrasana, Halasana (plough pose), Ardha Salbhasana, Salabhasana, (Locust) Bhujangasana, (1) Cobra pose, Vakrasana, Asana, Shavasana, (Relaxation) Yogamudra, Shirshasana (Head Stand) etc. These can be properly learnt under the guidance of experts. The Yoga lays down elaborate rules for maintaining the health of the body and making a fit vehicle for concentrated thought.

Pranayama is the regulation of breath. It consists in deep inspiration (Puraka), retension of breath (Kumbhaka) and expiration (Rechaka) with measured duration. It can also be learnt under the guidance of experts. That respiratory exercises are useful for strengthening the heart & improving its function is recognised by medical men when they recommend walking, climbing etc., in a graduated scale, for patients with weak hearts.

Tension and emotional stress, Insomnia, neurasthenia, fatigue, Indigestion, Backache and aching legs, lumbago and sciatica, Asthma, bronchitis, fever, Arthritis, gout, Rheumatism, obesity, female disorders, Headache, stiff neck, stomach, kidney and liver complaints, worries, cares and anxieties etc. are cured and Avarice, fear, anger etc. may be overcome by the Yogic practices.

Acupuncture, massage, zone therapy and Yoga nullify the doctrine of medicines and support the statement of Dr. Bellokossy.

The human organism is a store-house of energy. The practices of acupuncture, massage, zone therapy & yoga awaken or stimulate the imbalanced vital principle to take care of the store-house and run the divine creation smoothly for the higher purpose of existence.

These practices have made the science of crude medicines useless and Homoeopathy is not antagonistic to them because it also stimulates the vital principle by its subtle stimulus. They can work together without interfering the other & they may work as complementary to each other. So in case of Transmission of Homoeo drug energy, no drug as such is administered and a number of patients are recovering from various ailments and many are already cured. The author's discovery supports Dr. Bellokossy fully.

CHAPTER IV

THE DYNAMIC ACTION OF PLANTS FROM A DISTANCE

In the previous chapter we have seen how energy is supplied to the human organism by pricking needles and zone therapy. In this chapter it would be seen how ecology of the earth plays its role in our life. The culture of a country influences the art and science of healing. Not only the art of healing is influenced by the culture but also the organism is influenced by it. Even foetus is influenced by the environment when it is in the mother's womb by her emotions, food etc. When it first opens its eyes in the world, it is very much embarrassed by the outer world, which is quite different from the womb. From the very birth it is influenced by its environment, culture etc. Thus heredity and environment play a great role in modelling its character. The environment not only models its personality but also it is responsible for sound health. If it lives in a damp place, it gets sick by exposure. The plants, planets, the insects, the animal, all influence the persons who come in their contact. The experiments of Hydrogen and the Atom bombs have not done less harm to the humanity by their radiations.

Dr. Bankim Chandra Chatterjee has thrown a flood of light over the bad effects of explosion of bombs in his article "Radiation, Sickness & its Treatment" in "The Torch of Homoeopathy" January 1961, on page 5. He, in "Preliminary Report of the International Medical Commission of the effects on human health of Atomic & Hydrogen Bomb Explosion in Japan, 1955," says that the story of the atomic bomb explosions over Hiroshima and Nagasaki in early August, 1945 has passed into history. Since then other atomic bombs have been exploded experimentally and the development of the much more powerful thermonuclear hydrogen bomb has led to further experimental explosions, particularly at Bikini. The first explosion took place in March, 1954. It is sad to write here that our international experts say that there is no specific therapy for radiation sickness. It cannot be denied that they have effect on health. It can create total radiation diseases as well as diseases like anorexia, nausea, vomiting, diarrhoea, fever, mental disturbance, vertigo, loss of vision etc. It is not necessary that the explosions affected only those who are near the site but the whole world has been affected. It may be that the symptoms produced by radiations at greater distance may not be so.

The civilization is spoiling the air on the earth by artificial radiations and every moment we are breathing that polluted air from the atmosphere on one hand and the green mother earth is protecting from them and soothing us with her flora around us. Instinctively we are aware of the aesthetic radiations of plants. Plants and flowers have been the sources of inspiration and happiness in all walks of life from inception to the grave. Flowers are tokens of love and affection, of friendship or homage. Houses are decorated with them. Poets and philosophers all are delighted in the gardens and they have depicted them a paradise. Wordsworth enjoys immense pleasures while dancing with "Daffodils". Nature is not only a solace to human beings but it provides them with major portion of their food they consume every day. "All together 25 million square miles of leaf surface are daily engaged in this miracle of photosynthesis, producing oxygen and food for man and beast." "Of the 375 billion tons of food we consume each year, the bulk comes from plants."

Plants play vital role in every walk of life. They provide with bulk of medicines also. Mr. Bach believed that every living thing radiates and plants with high vibrations elevate the lower vibrations of human beings. Simoneton says that herbs, flowers, roots & barks have not only medicinal properties due to chemical contents but they radiate healthy wave lengths.

Plants emanate balmy radiations for the living beings. The author recollects his experiences of childhood in the rural areas, where radiation of plumb leaf is well known for a cure of stye on eye lids, when the author had stye on his eye lid, he was advised by the parents to hung plumb leaves just against the door of the house so that he could see them on walking up in the morning. The author followed their advice & in a couple of days he was free from stye. This practice is prevalent still to-day in the rural areas.

Another prevalent practice is to cure aphthae in the

mouth. The person having this trouble goes to a palm tree early in the morning and looking towards its top makes mouth to the tree. By so doing for some days he is free from that trouble. These practices so doing for some days he is free from that trouble. These practices are not baseless, rather they have reality and are based on the healthy radiations of plants.

Dr. B.N. Saxena, has devoted himself in studying dynamic action of the drugs and plants. He has cured innumerable patients suffering from chronic and acute ailments. It is not known what distance has been covered by radiation but it is a fact that the plants influence the patients from a distance. Let us hear learned Dr. Saxena in his own words which run in his article under the caption "The Dynamic Action of Drugs & Plants by their external exhibition from Distance", in "The Torch of Homoeopathy" January, 1961.

It is well-known that the dynamic power of the potentised Homoeopathic drugs set up a curative process in the vital force even when administered in very minute dose, touching the tongue or the nerve ending or skin surface and even by olfaction (smelling).

Hahnemann (Organon 6th Edition) has also acknowledged the homoeoathic curative effects of mesmerism, magnetism, will-force-and suggestive passes.

It is also known that various objects like colours, plants, metals, stones etc. affect the human physical and mental economy, when worn on body, and even kept in pockets.

All these led me to imagine that various plants influence the vital force or the economy of the human system even when exhibited from a distance. It was, however, borne in mind that different plants, roots, seeds, leaves, etc. may have different qualities and quantities of radiation with special effects on different organs of the human body. This thought led me to go deeper on the subject and experiments.

During the course of my research and experiments, I am amused to see that the exhibition of some of the plants to the sick persons even from a distance of a few feet or miles does exert some radiation of curative influence so that the patient can be relieved or cured of agonising pains, fevers etc. instantaneously.

The deeper I went into my researches and experiments, the more I was convinced of the tremendous powers of such radiation of plants. It may be difficult at present to explain the law of nature behind such phenomena in its full extent but it opens up a vast field of scientific research in ascertaining the peculiar virtues of each plant and its parts of their influences (or radiation effects) on sick persons by exhibition from distance, and the modes of exhibition such as brandishing, twisting, signalling, pressing upwards, downwards, backwards, sideways, times and measures of such exhibition etc. etc. because during the course of my researches and experiments I found that the same plant exhibited in different ways, produced different creative effects. This may have some conjoint effect of the spiritual powers and thoughts of the operator also which however, may also be borne in mind.

During the course of my researches and experiments with hundreds of plants and other drugs for the last 30 years, I have discovered the peculiar effects of some of the drugs and hence developed the process of exhibition or manipulation of the same for various curative purposes and am astounded with the miraculous results.

It is not possible to write all the details about all the plants and their manipulations in this small paper; but for your convenience I am giving below the summary of few such plants which stand out for their out standing effects on ailments of particular types and organs mentioned against each, so that you may start with the experiments forthwith with encouraging results:—

Name of plants	Organs and ailments
1. Shankh Pushpi	Navel
2. Sehdevi (Rohra fifdin Roxb)	Fever, Sunstroke etc.
3. Akra white (Calotropis Gigantica)	All sorts of fevers, sunstroke, Epilepsy, Teething etc.
4. Gunja (Beed tree & abrus-pricatorious Lill.)	Snake bite, delivery complications etc.
5. Saras (Mimesa Sarisa Roxb)	Teething complications, Snake bite, Sunstroke, Epilepsy.

6. Apamarg (achyranthus aspera)
All sorts of pains, eyesight, vertigo, burning sensation, high intermittent and bilious fevers, deafness etc.

7. Punarnava (Trismthema montgyma)
Jaundice, Enlarged liver or spleen Snake bite etc.

8. Mehdi
Insomnia, Heat, ulcers.

9. Dhatoora (Stramonium)
Habitual miscarriage, all sorts of fever.

10. Jalbhangra or Ghamra.
Malaria.

A test trial of the effects of the exhibition of such plants from distance was held before some scientists, at the instance of the Council of Scientific and Industrial Research, Government of India, New Delhi, who were impressed and so decided to cultivate some of the plants as per my suggestions in the National Botanical Garden, Lucknow.

Successful demonstrations were also held at the Government Ayurvedic College and Hospital, Jaipur, before the medical authorities. For the readers' interest, I give below a few cases treated by me recently at the Govt. Hospital, as specific instances.

1.   Date 31.8.60 : Patient, Laddoo Gopal, age 18, suffering from Earache (right ear) since 2 days. After examination he was given treatment. Noise was produced by loudly clapping (on applying juice of the plant Achyranthus aspera over the palms) near his right ear.

Result : Cured within 2 minutes. The pain had no relapse.

2.   Date 2.9.60 : Patient, Ramswaroop, age 13, suffering from pain in right leg & could hardly walk due to boil over his knee, even after 2 days treatment at the Hospital.

He was given treatment by me, by pressing the root of the plant Achyranthus aspera by both hands (right hand up) from a distance of about 2 ft. in front of the patient. Then pressed the root from 4 ft. and again from 6 ft.

The same action was repeated twice more, when the pain subsided and the patient could easily run about before the medical authorities — cured within 5 minutes. He was re-examined next day when he had absolutely no pain. The boil gradually subsided.

3.   Date 5.9.60 : Patient, Vinesh Chandra, age 14, student.

His right hand had a very slow growth since birth and as compared with his left hand, it looked about 40% thinner. It was deformed with stiff and bent fingers and the thumb due to which he could not clench the fingers into a fist.

The treatment was given by brandishing the twig of Achyranthus before him. The first day twice for 5 minutes each time, when 50% improvement was observed. Next day all his fingers and thumb were made to turn into a fist perfectly well and freely after repeating the said ction.

4.   Date 9.9.60 : Patient, Govind Ram, age 19, student. Stone deaf by left ear since 8 years and was declared incurable by Hospital authorities.

On examination by Earscope, his inner portion of left ear was found perforated and the ear base was lacerated and stinking with pus.

Treatment : Oiled the ear thrice at an interval of 20 minutes with plain Til oil.

The exhibition of the plant Achyranthus aspera was done thrice daily. Improvement was observed the first day and then there was improvement in hearing each day.

After treatment fo. 4 days he could hear a table calling bell from a distance of about 75 yards, also human voice clearly.

5.   Date 14.6.69 : Patient, Kishin Singh, age 28. Suffering from acute severe headache. Treatment was given by producing radiations through pressing the root of the plant Rohra Fifdin Roxb (Sehdevi) with both hands in front of the patient, cured immediately without any recurrence.

It is neither easy nor advisable to operate such treatment without being thoroughly acquainted with its methods by practical training.

However, I give below a few specific directions which can safely be experimented by any one in order to observe the strange, quick and curative effects on spot.

33   *Homoeo Drug Energy*

	Ailments	Prescribed drug	External mode of use
1.	Earache (acute pain in ear	Juice of Achyranthus aspera (use till it is fresh)	Apply on both palms and clap quickly a few times loudly.
2.	Disorder of the navel.	Shankh Pushpi (Plucked up on Monday)	Touch the root or twig over any sensitive part of the body for about 2 minutes.
3.	Bad eyesight of young age	Achyranthus aspera	Gazing at the root for about 30 seconds. Then get radiations from the root by swinging it before the patient and repeat this twice daily.
4.	Scorpion-bite	Gul Turra	Brandish the root a few times in front of the patient.
5.	Hemicrania	Adhasisi	Tie its seed with black thread at the ear on opposite side.
6.	Headache (acute pain)	Achyranthus aspera	Press the root with full strength before the patient by both hands from about 1 ft. Do so again from 2 ft. and then 3 ft. and repeat this action twice more.

A fair trial on the above lines alone may convince one and all of the dynamic effects of plants and drugs upon the vital force; even from a distance.

I believe, if the manipulation with these plants are properly studied and applied much curative results can be obtained even from a distance.

I invite students to learn what I have discovered with a

continued hard work for 30 years without any remuneration. I also invite the opinions and open minded criticism from the readers.

Dr. Chandra Prakash, the Editor of "Torch of Homoeopathy" has stated in his editorial note on page 4 of January, 61 issue, that one Dr. Saxena, recently demonstrated to us that some of the plants and roots have some power of radiation with their own peculiar virtues, so that the same may influence the sick person so favorable if properly applied even from a distance of several feet, that the patient immediately gets relief from his pains and cries turn into smiles within a fraction of second.

"He claims to have recognised such radiant powers of some 13 plants with their peculiar virtues to influence some diseased conditions. He claims that such radiation of some of these plants if exhibited from a distance of some feet or even several miles, can cure acute pains, high fevers of almost all types. He says than even some cases of blindness, deafness, paralysis etc. can also be cured with continued treatment for a short period but not from great distance".

"Out of these 13 plants, he told us, Achyranthus Aspera (Apmarg or Apaang) is one, which, if exhibited to the patient from a distance, and twisted in particular manner, can relieve the patients of various pain and fevers almost instantaneously. We know the various Homoeopathic uses of Achyranthus and we know that by the law of nature the homoeopathic medicines work in infinitesimal dose; hence it should not be difficult for us to believe that such powerful drugs may act by radiation from a distance".

We also know that some sensitive persons are allergic to some plants so that they develop physical and mental symptoms even if they pass by near those plants. Some plants like Rhus Tox. affect almost every body more or less even from distance.

"Knowledge that does not generate achievement is a pale and bloodless thing unworthy of mankind".

"So what I pray is that let us also not fall prey to dogmatism. The fundamental laws of Homoeopathy have been well tried, applied and proved again and again for the last 160 years and there cannot be any dispute over that. Those who condemn them today for their own ignorance without proper trial are themselves the sufferers and losers. But let us not fight with anybody, let us preach the laws of nature or the truth as much as known to us and prove it by cures of sick persons. The readers who care will gradually learn and benefit from exchange of knowledge and experience".

Homoeopathy has a sound philosophy behind the science with fundamental laws of cure, co-ordinating the knowledge of the body, mind, soul, vital force etc. in health and sickness and the causes of diseases and effect of drugs and their actions and reactions in various forms.

Let us go ahead and seek further if we meet with such truth which may be co-ordinated with our science and art of Homoeopathy for the purpose of the highest ideal of curing the sick by "rapid, gentle, and permanent restoration of health by removal and annihilation of the disease in its whole extent, in the shortest, most reliable and most harmless way, on easily comprehensible principles".

Hahnemann has referred to the curative effects of magnetism, mineral magnets, electricity, galvanism, mesmerism, baths etc. and has said that they are also homoeopathic (L 266 to 291 Organon 6th edition) or act as palliative or partly as homoeopathic serviceable aid etc.

Thus he opened a way for his followers to go deeper and further in the study of these subjects for their systematic and scientific application, if possible and such other aids which may prove beneficial or helpful to achieve our end of ideal cure.

Many of the readers must have heard and seen some instances of faith cure, which is neither magic nor illusion. This also works with a law of nature but it might need more systematic study and practice to apply the law effectively for rapid, gentle and permanent cure.

I have seen some country folk curing appendicitis, colic, liver, dropsy, squint, rheumatism etc., by some gentle notes on the veins at the joints; and the cure is rapid, gentle, permanent and must be according to some law of nature which is not easily comprehensible to us because we do not and did not care to investigate.

Dr. B.N. Saxena is over 86 years and lives at Ajmer, Rajasthan at present. He is a medical officer and running a charitable dispensary there. He has trained a number of students on this line and he is continuing his philanthropic activities by educating students on this line and helping the poor by treatment. He calls his method of treatment "Medico Psycho-therapy".

His theory is based on philosophical, psychological as well as on the scientific thoughts. He states that while aiming at healation of the ailing persons by pressing, moving or brandishing the root or twigs of other plant concerned with its piece in hand by the healer, it radiates the impulses packed with dynamic force of healing energy from the plants' piece in the hand to the indisposed part of the ailing person through the atmosphere or Ether, eliminating the factors of space or length of distance and time. It causes the sensitive nerves to affect the heart sphere probably through the brain with a slight movement for regular functioning and giving response to healthy blood with the magnetic energy assisting the dynamic healing power to recoup the loss of energy of the affected organism causing quick healation through functioning of nervous system in every organ, affecting rapid, gentle, and permanent cure.

When the creation of these radiations is the result of the above actions with the plants' twig acted upon or displayed by the skilled operator and supported by the pushing of the will power through concentration, the same accelerates their velocity and effect the aimed target safer and quicker also effective to the mark than in ordinary cases related above.

Will power of the person is stronger in concentration of mind implies, that he has got only one state over his mental Retina to the exclusive of others. That one mental state is pressed with all force by the supreme will power at a speed velocity of heart and mind waves ranging from 4000 to 800000000000000 miles per second as compared with the speed of the light waves, wireless waves, electromagnetic waves and electric currents at 186000 miles per second, sound in air velocity at 1100 ft. per second, sound in water at 4400 ft. and in iron, velocity is at 17600 ft. per second only.

As regards the effects obtained through mental concentration at a preappointed time from distant places, it has enough similarity to connecting Radiograms, wherein the concerning values have to be adjusted in order to connect the particular hearing from different wavelengths.

Dr. Saxena also has observed that time is an important

factor in case of Dynamic radiations of plants. It is observed that certain plants uprooted at particular time provide miraculous results. This is because of the fact that the movement of certain planets of the earth in particular design of walks forming change in seasons, spring and autumn, summer, winter and rainy seasons, brings a turn to the entire substance of the universe, providing changing effects in herbs and plants. It adds more energy to the dynamic force of healing in herbs and plants during full moon, solar and lunar eclipses or at other times and Nakshatras, in other words when the earth is awake. If uprooted within the said periods, the energetic power remains preserved with the plants, otherwise it leaks away back to the mother earth with change of stars' influence. Such plants have to be preserved from the sun rays which snatch away their created energy and saved from being touched with the iron metal, the same being detrimental to their mercurial properties rendering the plants weak for healing purpose.

Besides the cases noted above Dr. Saxena has cured various patients by his "Medico Psychotherapy" from a distance. The three cases treated by him through phone are worth mentioning. It is reported that through phone from Delhi, immediate relief was observed in cases of Railway officials suffering from lumbago and chest pain at Rawan & Bantikui at a distance of 52 miles and 125 miles respectively as a result of the actions with the drugs.

Further it is added that a result of druggic actions from Abu Road without a connecting medium instantaneous and prompt relief was observed to the sickly daughter of Sri N.K. Durgapal, M.A.C.T., Railway High School, Abu Road.

After the recovery of his daughter whose life was in danger Sri Durgapal granted a testimonial to Dr. Saxena which reads as follows :—

"I believe in the healing power of the drugs through Medico psychotherapy—a treatment done through performing certain physical action with the help of the drugs from a distance. It is all the more astonishing that even long distance makes no difference into this method of divine treatment."

Dr. B.N. Saxena is a great devotee to the science of healing. He is energetic and he possesses untiring zeal to further the art of healing. It transpires from the method of his treatment that he has combined drug energy and plants' radiations with psychology. From the very heading of his method of treatment (Medico-Psychotherapy), it appears that he has confused drug action with mental phenomena. No doubt he has cured innumerable cases by his method but the readers will find that there is no clear distinction whether plants' radiation or mental concentration is prominent in handling. However, from the above statements it is clear that transmission of drugs and plants is possible in curing patients from a distance.

CHAPTER V

TREATMENT THROUGH PHOTOGRAPH

In the aforesaid Chapters, we have seen how Homoeopathic medicines influence the persons in health or sickness from a distance. In this Chapter, it will be shown how Cosmic Rays or drug energy is transmitted to the sick from a distance, through photograph.

Before going in details as to how Cosmic Rays are being transmitted, let us analyses the very constitutions of organism and creations of the world of matter and mind.

Science, Arts, Philosophy, Metaphysics, Astronomy etc. influence the culture of a country and in its turn it influences them. The art and science of Medical Therapy is not an exception.

The human beings are born and brought up in the lap of Nature, speaking in a broader sense and they earn their livelihood, pass their days and breathe their last in the end. They are very much surprised to see the various beautiful scenes as well as the angry mood of Nature. They enjoy and suffer and try to get rid of sufferings. They devise means to bring their sufferings to an end by discovering medical arts, crude or fine. The Indian Philosophy starts from the very idea to get rid of sufferings by real knowledge as ignorance is the root cause of all sufferings. To know the truth means to know the real nature of the Natural Phenomena which give births to different sciences, arts etc. Different approaches are made to know according to the levels of achievement in the different fields. In ancient times in our country or abroad in the undeveloped parts of the world specially the primitive societies and other backward communities the approach to life was quite different from the developed societies. In the field of Medicine we see different approaches— Witch-craft, Tantras, Mantras & other superstitious beliefs are prevalent to cure ailing beings, but there is a tinge of truth everywhere. Human knowledge is limited and efforts are being made to unravel the mysteries of Nature. Nature is inspiration as well as the source of knowledge. It is the major premise from which all the conclusions are derived rightly or wrongly. The healing art also draws its conclusion from its appearance or parts of it, but the natural whole is beyond comprehension uptil now. This is just like an elephant for a blind man who bases his definition of the elephant by touching a particular part of it, but his statement is not wholly wrong.

The Naturopath treats patients by natural phenomena like earth, water, light etc. It is mainly based on 5 elements of nature. The Biochemistry of Dr. Schuessler finds remedies in twelve salts only which are called "Tissue Remedies". Among the tribes and other undeveloped societies crude practices in the realm of Therapeutics are in vogue. When a patient is suffering from high blood pressure or high temperature, the head is broken to let blood out to release the tension of the brain or leach is applied to suck the so-called bad blood. The modern highly developed orthodox school of Medicines also punctures the lumber of the delirious patients to bring the spinal fluid out to reduce tension of the brain.

The Ayurvedic system of treatment has been very much influenced by the Vedas, rather it has originated from the great scriptures, the Vedas and bases its principles on Triads, i.e. three Principles—Cough, Pitta and Vata. The Indian system of treatment is very much influenced by its Philosophy and Meta-physics.

1.   The Cosmic Rays Therapy

The late Dr. B. Bhattacharya of Naihaty was the exponent of "The Cosmic Rays Therapy." Marvellous cures have been reported by him in his Book, "The Science of Cosmic Rays Therapy". This system is based on the seven colours of Nature. It has been influenced by our ancient Metaphysics particularly "The Sankhya" system. To understand this, it will not be out of place to throw light on this system.

The Sankhya system deals with dualism—two realities— Prakriti and Purusa. Its Metaphysics is based mainly on the theory of Causation which we are concerned with. According to its causation means a real transformation of the Cause into the effect which logically leads to the concept of Prakriti as the ultimate cause of the creation of the objects of the world. All the objects of the world, including own body, mind, the senses and the intellect are dependent and united as they are produced by the combination of elements. The Prakriti manifests itself in different forms by the influence of Purusa. At the time of destruction all the objects are resolved into physical elements and the latter into atoms, the atoms into energies and so on, till all the products are resolved into the unmanifested eternal Prakriti which is a unity in diversity. In case of creation the process is reverse. The Science of to-day also holds the view that matter is energy and energy is matter, i.e. matter is resolved into energy and vice versa.

Prakriti is constituted by the three gunas of Sattva, Rajas and Tamas. It is equilibrium. Guna is a constituent element or substance, not an attribute. The three gunas are like the strands of the same rope. In our daily life we observe that everything of the world has got three gunas. As for example, the cuckoo's cry is pleasant to the beauty-loving artist, painful to the sick and neither to the simple rustic. Sattva is that element of Prakriti which is of nature of pleasure. It is bright or illuminating. Rajas is the principle of activity or dynamism in things. It is the cause of all unpleasant experiences. Tamas is the principle of passivity and negativity in things. It has the nature of indifferences. Hence Sattva, Rajas and Tamas have been compared to whiteness, redness and darkness. These gunas are in the state of both conflict and co-operation with each other. The classification of objects into good, bad and indifferent or into pure, impure and neutral or into intelligent, active and dolent is based on dominance of Sattva, Rajas and Tamas respectively. Another characteristic of the gunas is that they are constantly changing or transforming.

With the contact between Purusa and Prakriti, there is a disturbance of equilibrium in which gunas were held together before the creation. Rajas being active is disturbed first. This produces a tremendous commotion in the unfathomable womb of Prakriti and each of the gunas tries to preponderate over each other. Out of chaos there is cosmos.

The first product of the evolution of Prakriti is the "Buddhi" or intellect and the second is "Ahankara" or the ego.

Ahankar is said to be of three kinds—Sattvika, Rajasa & Tamasa. From Sattvika arise eleven organs-the five sensory organs and the five organs of actions, and the mind. From Tamasa the five subtle elements are derived. The second is concerned with both to supply energy. The five subtle elements are genetic essences of sound, touch, colour, taste and smell. These are very subtle and can not be perceived by the sensory organs. The five subtle elements give birth to five gross physical elements.

Akash (ether) is produced from the essence of sound with a quality of sound which is perceived by the ear. Air is produced from the essence of touch combined with that of sound which has the attributes of sound and touch. From the essence of colour (form) mixed with those of sound and touch arises fire or light with attributes of sound, touch and colour. Water is produced from the essence of taste combined with those of sound, touch and colour with the qualities of sound, touch, colour and taste. In the same way smell is produced from the essence of smell combined with those of sound, touch, colour (form) taste and smell. The human organism is constituted from the above elements plus self (soul) the very essence of consciousness. The latter portion does not come in our purview here.

From the above accounts it is clear why certain elements come in the domain of therapy. Colour plays its role in the therapy of cosmic rays. Ailments arise out of deficiency of different colours in the body. There are seven colours "VIBG-YOR" which maintain the qualities of health. On this principle the use of stone has important role in curing ailments and different planets influence the organism. Each planet represents colour. The following table will give an idea of days, planets and colour:—

"Day	Planet	Colour-Symbol	
Sunday	Sun	Red-	R.
Monday	Moon	Orange-	O.
Tuesday	Mars	Yellow-	Y.
Wednesday	Mercury	Green-	G.
Thursday	Jupiter	Blue-	B.
Friday	Venus	Indigo-	I.
Saturday	Saturn	Violet-	V."

"Element	Principle Rudements	Sensory Organs	Cosmic Colour Rays
Akash	Sound	Ears	Blue
Air	Touch	Skin	Violet
Fire	Form	Eyes	Red
Water	Taste	Tongue	Orange
Earth	Smell	Nose	Green"

The above accounts of evolution of the world may be compared with the atomic theory.

The three gunas represent the Tridosh of Ayurveda— Vayu,Pitta and Cough, and neutral, negative and positive of science. The following table will make it clear:—

Gunas	Forces	Doshas	Element
Sattva	Harmony(Neutral)	Vayu	Akash & Air
Rajasa	Energy (Negative)	Pitta	Fire
Tamasa	Inertia(Positive)	Cough	Water & Earth

Rings with different stones (gems) are used according to the advice of the experts in the line to cure sufferings caused due to the influence of different planets. This table will give a clear idea.

Gems	Planets	Rays
Ruby	Sun	Red
Pearl	Moon	Orange
Coral	Mars	Yellow
Emerald	Mercury	Green
Moonstone	Jupiter	Blue
Diamond	Venus	Indigo
Sapphire	Saturn	Violet
Sardonyx	Rahu	Ultraviolet
Cat's, eye	Ketu	Infrared."

Dr. Bhattacharya in his book, "The Science of Cosmic Rays Therapy" has given in details how Cosmic Rays are transmitted to cure different ailments. The rays is transmitted through the medium of a photograph of the patient. It is said that the photograph has got the same wave length which the patient has. If cosmic rays are applied on the photograph, they travel on the same wave length and affect the patient at a distance. The photograph is examined with the help of a prism. The nose of the photograph of the patient is viewed through a prism. If the colour of the nose is different from that of a healthy person, it means that the person needs certain Rays. According to the requirement of colour, gems are selected and fixed in a disk which is fitted in a table fan. The photograph is fixed infront of the fan and the switch of the fan is made on to rotate throwing the rays of the gems over the photograph for certain time and changes take place in colour of nose and then again, the nose is viewed through the prism. If the nose shows normal colour then the process is stopped and the patient at distant place is cured simultaneously.

Number of rays differs from month to month and the following table shows these variations.

"SPACE OF THE COSMIC RAYS"

"Sign	Months with dates	No. of Rays
Capricorn	15th Jan. to 14th February	5000
Aquarius	15th Feb. to 14th March	6000
Pisces	15th March to 14th April	7000
Aries	15th April to 14th May	8000
Taurus	15th May to 14th June	9000
Gemini	15th June to 14th July	10000
Cancer	15th July to 14th August	10000
Leo	15th August to 14th September	11000
Virgo	15th Sept. to 14th October	10000
Libra	15th Oct. to 14th November	8000
Scorpion	15th November to 14th December	7000
Sagittarius	15th Dec. to 14th January	6000

Particular rays are required to cure particular diseases.

The following diseases require Red Rays:—"Old age infirmity, T.B., Colic, Constipation, Insanity, Goiter, Obesity, Collapse, Asthma, High Blood Pressure, Cancer, Sleeplessness, Idiocy, Worms, Sleepiness and all Cough and vayu diseases etc."

2. "Orange Rays are required for burning sensation of various parts, Fissures, Syphilis, Rheumatic Heart, loss of sperm,

bleeding, epilepsy, Convulsions, Cancer due to vitiated blood, Bleeding piles, Indigestion etc."

3. "Yellow Rays are needed in Dropsy, Constipation, Enlargement of liver and spleen, lumbago, urticaria, dry cough, Piles due to Vayu, Asthma, Obesity, Insanity, Anaemia, Impotency, fever, all cough diseases etc.

4.   Green Rays cure "Ozaena, Cholera, Skin disease, aphonia, bleeding piles, Retension of urine, Swelling, Tumour, Abortions, Anaemia, Small Pox; all pitta diseases etc."

5.   Blue Rays cure "Syphilis, Nausea, Vomiting, Hysteria, Diarrhoea, Bleeding Piles, Insanity, Scorpion bite, effects of poison, whooping cough, all Vayu diseases etc."

6.   Indigo Rays are said to cure "Indigestion, Cough, Piles due to Cough, Hiccough, Fever, Epilepsy, Fistula, all pitta diseases etc."

7.   Diseases requiring violet Rays:—"Pains, Hardness and roughness, colic, gas, Paralysis, Hiccough, Palpitation, Speechlessness, Hysteria, Mental diseases, Ulcers, all Vayu diseases, etc."

Now the readers are fully acquainted with the above method of treatment. Dr. Bhattacharya claims to have cured various ailments of human being as well as of animals by this therapy.

This method has got various merits:—(1) Treatment is possible even in absence of the patient, simply by sending his photograph. It is said that even the handwriting and clothes of the patients may be used as medium. (2) By this method diagnosis of a cisease is made by examining the photograph through the prism. (3) and the patients have not to bother to take medicines etc. (4) The Doctor could know the progress without examining the patients.

No doubt, this method has the above merits but it is cumbersome to handle. From the above accounts it is obvious that treatment in space is possible by transmitting the cosmic rays through the medium of a photograph of the patient at distant places, hence distance is no bar. The patients need not take oral medicines, i.e. taking medicine is not essential in curing ailments.

2.   Broadcasting of Radionic Pesticides

A French Engineer, Mr. Andre Simoneton's imagination that one day the physicians with earphones would diagnose patients simply by tuning into the frequencies emitted from the sick or their diseased organs and then cure them by broadcasting healthy Vibrations is no more a fiction now. We have already seen in the Previous Chapter how Dr. Albert Abrams detected human radiations and utilised them for diagnosis of a disease. The omnipresent electromagnetic waves are incident from all directions on infinite number of planes. We, all are bathing in their fields and are being influenced by them every moment. There is a close relationship between the geomagnetic field and the electromagnetic fields of individuals. Working in this field Dr. Abrams could pin-point a particular disease at a particular organ. The age-long concept that a disease was of a cellular origin was given a forceful blow by replacing it by molecular constituents of cells. He could diagnose the ailments of the human body with his instrument simply from a single drop of his blood. According to him all matter is radioactive and the waves can be picked up in space by using human "reflexes" as detectors.

Mr. Curtis P. Upton, a Princeton-trained Civil Engineer went on to think if he could use the strange device meant for curing human ailments in the field of Agriculture to control pest. In 1951, he, along with his classmate, William J. Knuth, an electronic expert from Corpus Christi, Texas went into the Cotton field for experiments. They wanted to affect the field through its photograph hence they took an aerial photograph of the field. The photograph was placed on the Collector Plate attached to the base of the instrument about the size of a portable radio, together with a reagent known to be poisonous to cotton pests. The dials were set in a specific manner. The aim of the experiment was to clear the field of pests without using Costly Chemical insecticides. The theory behind the system—as "way out" as anything so far reported on the nature of plants— held that the molecular and atomic makeup of the emulsion on the photograph would be resonating at the identical frequencies of the objects they represented pictorially. By affecting the photograph with a reagent known to be poisonous to cotton pests the Americans believed the cotton plants in the field could be immunized against pests." The amount of the poisonous reagent was used in infinitesimal dosages thinking that it would act in the same way as Homoeopathic diluted medicines do. The device was used for pest control, which increased the cotton yield by 25% per acre over the state average as the Tucson "Week-end-Reporter" reported. It was also reported that the area exposed to this strange treatment was free from snakes.

"On the East Cost of the United States, one of the Upton's Princeton Classmates, Howard Armstrong, who had become an industrial chemist with many inventions to his credit, decided to try his friend's method in Pennsylvania. After taking an aerial photograph of a corn field under attack by Japanese beetles, he cut one corner off the photo with a pair of scissors and laid the remainder together with a small amount of rotenone, a beetle poison, extracted from the roots of a Woody Asia Vine which the Japanese call "roten" on the Collector plate of one of Upton's radionic devices."

"After several five-to ten-minute treatments with the machine's dial set to specific readings, a meticulous count of beetles revealed that 80-90 percent of them had died or disappeared from the corn plants treated through the photo. The untreated plants in the corner cut away from the photo remained 100 percent infested.

This experiment is very thrilling & revealing. It should have been encouraged & experimented for the benefit of the human race but instead of giving credit it was turned down taking it as unreal, fantastic & crazy even after witnessing this experiment. The people go by the preconceived notions.

According to De La warr "each molecule of matter is capable of producing a tiny electrical voltage that is a specific to itself, and which transmits' rather like a tiny radio transmitter-receiver. A collection of molecules therefore, is capable of transmitting a generic pattern. This means that the signal from a plant or human is quite individual, and that each plant or person will receive a transmission on their own generic pattern. It is here that the photograph plays its part, as it is thought that the emulsion on the negative retains the generic pattern of the object photographed & can be induced to reradiate as a carrier. Thus, with a photograph of a plant in circuit it is possible to affect that plant at a distance".

The incident of 1955-56 of a tribal village of Ranchi is still fresh in mind. Some visitors came to see the works done under the Community Development programmes in the tribal areas. They were ignorant of their customs, taboos, beliefs etc. and without meaning anything they look the photograph of the tribal people called Oraon. The villagers were very furious on this act and rushed to attack them. However, they took to their heels & the villagers were somehow pacified by us. On enquiry it was learnt that they have are-long-honoured belief that by photography their lives would be shortened or their souls would be captured. Whatever may be their belief but it is a fact that the photograph has close relationship with the person or object photographed. The photograph has the same frequency as that of the individual person or plant and it can be used as a good medium for transmitting drug energy to cure the suffering humanity as well as other living beings.

3. Homoeo Drug Transmission

In the very beginning of the author's discovery of "TRANS-MISSION OF HOMOEO DRUG ENERGY FROM A DISTANCE" through a detached hair of the patient, it was assumed that any natural belonging to the patient may be used for the purpose. Some experiments on blood, signature, handwriting, voice even photo etc. were done successfully but hair is very handy and convient that is why it has been used in practices.

The above experiment of Howard Armstrong in the field of agriculture induced the author to try Homoeo drug on the photograph of the patient. The result was wonderful hence all the Research Scholars of the "Research Institute of Sahni Drug Transmission & Homoeopathy were asked to experiment & report. The author himself made the following experiments:—

Case No. 1—The first experiment was done on the author's youngest son, Pradeep Kumar Sahni, who had no trouble at the time of experiment. One globule of N. V. 200 was placed at his photograph & after 2 minutes he experienced pain in head. The globule was removed from the photograph & head-ache vanished atonce. Again it was transmitted through it & headache re-appeared along with tingling sensation & pain in the lower extremities. Finally the globule was removed & pain along with tingling vanished atonce.

Case No. 2—Master S. Nath aged 19 had headache which

was aggravated by motion. One globule of Bry. 200 was placed at his photograph at a distance of 5 k.m. His headache vanished atonce & he felt afresh. The globule was removed finally.

Case No. 3—Mrs. S. Nath aged 50 had pain in eyes, Chest & shoulders. She has phone in her house at a distance of 5 k.m. from the author's Chamber. One globule of N.V. 200 was placed at her photograph & she atonce felt urge for stool & went to the latrine, pain vanished & violent itching started at the site of pain. She began to belch continuously. Then the globule was removed from the photograph, & itching & belching subsided.

Case No. 4—The subject of Case No. 1 having electric shock on 21-7-77, had pain in head, upper & lower extremities. One pill of Phos 0/12 was placed at his photograph. Pain in lower extremities aggravated first & extended to thighs also. Pain & indisposition completely disappeared after 15 minutes & the pill was removed.

Case No. 5—Master Deepak Kumar Shrivastava aged 14 years, son of Shri M.L. Shrivastava fell ill. He had temperature, diarrhoea, Vomiting & Colic from 18-7-77. He was treated by Dr. S. Sahni, (the author's wife). He had been free from all troubles by noon of 21-7-77 but fever & diarrhoea relapsed from the evening.

On enquiry it was learnt that his pet parrot died in the morning of 18-7-77 which was just like a bolt from the blue. Taking grief as the cause of troubles, one globule of Ignatia 200 was placed at his photograph on 21-7-77. The result was miraculous. He began to feel better and by the morning of 22-7-77 he was free from all troubles.

Here is a report by Dr. R.K.P. Sinha on his experiments:—
I have been treating patients by Homoeopathic medicines through transmission since long. Recently I was directed by the director R.I.S.D.T. to experiment transmission through photographs. It could be done only with those cases whose photographs were available and naturally I chose my own family for it.

Case No. 6—"On 25-6-77, my wife complained to me that she had a sprain in her right ankle. I put a drop of Rhus. Tox. 30 (diluted in water) on her photograph. (The photograph was a group family photograph). No sooner I dropped the medicine on the photograph she felt improvement in pain. At that time I could not think out as to how to continue the transmission with the photograph and she got well in course of the day".

Case No. 7—"Next time on 29-6-77 my daughter Seema aged twelve years got her finger burnt while cooking. I used the same group family photograph, in which she also figured, for transmission. I put a drop of diluted Cantharis 30 and immediately she felt a feeling of coolness at the burnt spot. I allowed the drop to remain on the photograph till it got evaporated and she also did not feel the pain afterwards."

Treatment through photograph is not so convenient and handy as through hair. A drop of drug in the tincture form evaporates soon. Globule too needs special arrangement for preservation. The photograph of a patient may not be readily available.

PART-II

TRANSMISSION OF DRUG-ENERGY
THROUGH DETACHED HAIR OF PATIENT

CHAPTER I
TRANSMISSION OF DRUG-ENERGY THROUGH DETACHED HAIR OF PATIENT

1. Introduction

Ever since the discovery of Homoeopathic system of medicines by Samuel Hahnemann, the principle of *Similia similibus curenter* has remained unchanged and will never change as long as this system of medicine exists. Although the powerful force of electro-magnetic energy hidden inside each tiny globule of Homoeopathic medicine, has well been recognised and applied throughout the world, it is not justified to say that this system is static and no further improvement is possible. It has been evolving like an organism. This system of healing is eternal and Divine.

Everything of the world has got life within. It has consciousness latent in it. Even the stone has got latent consciousness as in the living body of man which is the most complex of Divine creation. The Homoeopathic medicine is dynamic. The globule, sugar of milk or alcohol is nothing but vehicle, a carrier and a body. It is material, non-medicinal and non-dynamic but the potentised medicine is immaterial. It is spiritual and vital. This soul-like entity should not be essentially a commodity to be taken orally. It is consciousness latent in matter (Aurobindo). There is a hierarchy in the scales of consciousness or vibration.

The problem of matter, mind and spirit has been confronting us since long. Matter is the subject matter of the materialist while consciousness is that of the idealist. The former gives emphasis on one aspect of the problem, while the other on the other aspect. But Hahnemann firmly putting his feet on the ground and his head in the heaven studied Man as an organism possessing vital principle within. For him matter, mind and vital principle are all realities and he made Homoeopathic science a meeting ground of physical science and metaphysics.

He knew the limitation of modern science. "The chemist guided by the law of chemical affinity and molecular attraction, reaches the sphere of Universal Attraction. He stops and turns away. The biologist, tracing life back through organism to the cell, and still further back to the formless bit of protoplasm lying as it were, on the shore of the infinite ocean of his life, also halts and turns away. The physicist analyses matter, divides and subdivides it until it disappears in the hypothetical, inanimate, unintelligent ether of space which he conceives to be the source both of matter and force, and there he also halts. Each is unsatisfied and must ever remain so until like Hahnemann, he yields to that innermost urge of the soul which demands of every man that he takes the final step and acknowledges the Infinite Life and Mind of the Universe, the source and substance of all power, the Father Eternal, to whom he owes spiritual allegiance."

Man is not only a combination of body and mind but has got something transcendental within him. He has vitality working within, as the vital principle is the cause of creation. It is working in the whole universe. The human organism is in its living state, a complete and integral whole. Every sensation, every manifestation of force (vitality) is inter-related. No part can suffer without involving all the rest. All things have individual influence having Aura around them. The process of two-way-traffic is found everywhere. There is a close relationship between the geomagnetic field and the electromagnetic fields of individuals. Human organism being unique, stands in relation to all parts of the universe in a constant action and reaction. It is unity, a harmony in diversity. But there is a hierarchy in the scales of life, vibration and susceptibility.

Man being a rational animal has animality as well as rationality within him. He tries to obtain sensual pleasures but is he satisfied with them ? Never, he tries to find out something transcendental shaking off his bondage. He tries to attain existence-consciousness-bliss which is the summum bonum of life. But he is confronted by diseases, physical, mental as well as spiritual, which are the counter-currents of vital force. Hence disease is also dynamic which is troubling the humanity. Homoeo. Dynamic medicines help the humanity by freeing him not only from bodily sufferings but also from mental and spiritual. Homoeopathy helps humanity in attaining his goal. The author does not want to be lost in the metaphysical problem of body, life, mind and soul. He can only say that they are inter-related in different planes of susceptibility.

The subtle nature of the Homoeopathic dynamic medi-cines led the author think about the tremendous electromag-netic energy hidden in a tiny globule of dynamic medicine which is radiating incessantly and possibility of finding out any medium through which this store-house of energy may be channelized in curing the suffering humanity. Radio wave can be transmitted and thought wave can be transmitted in the case of Tele-therapy, then why not this subtle energy of Homoeopa-thic dynamic medicine can be transmitted in space to cure ailing human beings ?

The problem as to how to transmit the Homoeopathic Dynamic Drug-Energy to the ailing human beings had been taxing the author's mind since long. He had no sleep during the night of 5.1.1967 due to the vexing problem in his mind. In the morning of 6.1.1967 Mr. A. Kumar of Bhagalpur came to him for the 2nd time to show his son, Master Pramod Kumar, a student of standard VIII of St. Xavier's H. E. School, Sahebganj, Santal Pragana, who had been suffering from eczema and examined by him on 26.12.1966. After repertorising the case by Kent's Repertory Ars. Alb. was selected and it was administered orally in 200th potency. Mr. A. Kumar himself, a patient of chronic peptic ulcer had been under the Ayurvedic treatment of Dr. R.C. Shastri who was absent that day. He requested him to give some medicine to get relief of his acute colic pain. A flash came to the author's mind to try Ars. Alb. 200 on his uprooted hair. Ars. Alb. was selected at random, as sometimes the same remedy helps the blood relations. He requested him to give a hair from his head and it was done. It was placed on the cover of a book and one globule of Ars. Alb. 200 was brought in contact with the root of his hair. Mr. Kumar uttered, "I am feeling a churning sensation in my abdomen". The author's joy knew no bounds. He detached the hair from the medicated globule and pain was reduced to 75% at once. He was very conscious of psychology at that time. He said, "Well the remaining 25% pain will vanish this time". Instead of using Ars. Alb. 1M he came down to 30th potency and one drop of it was poured on the root of the same hair. To utter surprise, the pain became so intense that he left his chamber in agony.

The cup of his joy was full to the brim as the long-standing taxing problem was solved.

He wrote down an article under the caption, "Homoeo Dynamic Medicines can be transmitted", which was published in the "Torch of Homoeopathy", April 1967 issue, New Colony, Jaipur, Rajasthan with encouraging comments and suggestions by the editor, Dr. Chandra Prakash Jhunjhunwala. Some books and articles were suggested by him to go through.

On 30.3.1967 Mr. A. Kumar, when he came to the author for his son, narrated that after going from him on 6.1.67 he had become almost unconscious due to intense colic and an allopathic physician was called in for his rescue. He had been confined to bed for a couple of days. But that was the last and most violent attack. He was relieved of his colic after three days and since then he had been free from his obstinate colic.

The 6th Jan. 1967 and Mr. A. Kumar will remain commemorable in the history of DISCOVERY OF TRANSMISSION OF DRUG-ENERGY THROUGH DETACHED HAIR OF PATIENT.

After this miraculous effect on Sri Kumar, the author had been awaiting for further experiment. The same day an old patient suffering from epilepsy came to the author & Lachesis 200 was transmitted in the above manner. Immediately the patient felt a current like sensation in his left arm for some seconds. Taking the remedy for correct one it was administered orally. In this way the author has been devoting his time in thinking & experimenting with success. According to the suggestions of Dr. Chandra Prakash Jhunjhunwala, the author collected the books and articles on the allied subjects and went through them to find out explanation as to how Drug energy is transmitted through hair already detached from the body but no answer was found out. Some of their topics were included in the first part of the book.

In the preceding chapters it has been narrated that some advances have been made in this field in various countries. Many of the research minded doctors, have taken considerable pains in finding out improvements particularly in the method of application of this system. Between 1914 and 1920 the late Dr. Albert Abrams of San Francisco made certain medico-physical discoveries of far reaching importance. He was one of the first physicians to turn his attention towards wireless waves which emanate from the human body. Dr. Boyd constructed an accurate apparatus called Emanometer for detecting the disease emanations and the corresponding drug-relation. Dr. Guyon Richard's research embraces the fields of Homoeopathy, radiesthesia, physics and metaphysics. Dr. John A. Hobbs and D. Henshaw threw a flood of light on radiesthesia or Radionic diagnosis. Dr. G.W. Boericke has studied, "Lipoid Flocculation Test" for the selection of Homoeopathic medicines. These advances have been made towards the diagnostic aspect of the problem only.

It has been seen how Dr. Saxena is engaged in studying dynamic action of the drugs and plants. He claims quite successful cures in a number of cases he treated. Plants influence the patients from a distance. Dr. Bhattacharya of Naihati had practised cosmic Rays-Therapy successfully in treating the patients by transmitting Cosmic rays through the medium of a photograph of the patient. These scientists have, no doubt, made excellent contributions in opening a new horizon of thought but the manner of application seems to be cumbersome.

2.   Is It Psychological ?

Again the question "How" began to tax the brain. Some people say that the effect of transmission on the patient is only psychological. No doubt, psychology plays a very important role in curing diseases particularly mental. Suggestions are given by the psychologists to the mental patients and their hidden emotions are brought from the depth of mind to the surface and in so-doing they get better. Even gout, Neuralgia etc. have been cured by psychoanalysis. We have seen in the preceding chapter how psychology has been mixed up with plants' radiations. The author was very particular on this point. Even while experimenting on the first case of Ars. Alb. he was cautious enough to guard this phenomenon. The objective and subjective effects have been observed very minutely on different age-groups of human beings as well as on mute animals. The medicine-energy has been transmitted on newly-born babies as well as on cows, cat, buffalo and dogs successfully. Even during sleep, effects have been observed. Hence emphatically, it can be said that the effects of transmission on the patients is never psychological.

3.   Is It Telepathy ?

The "guessing" of the thought linked with specific physio-
logical reactions of definite location, whether this "guessing"
rests on a rational process following on the observation of
reactions or on an intuitive faculty, presents as with something
which is not only kinetic, dynamic and quantitative, but also
qualitative and interpretative of emotional and mental states of
feeling. Telepathy is the word indicated by such facts. In the
word of F.W.H. Myers the term Telepathy means, "The communication of impressions of any kind from one minded to another,
independently of the recognised channels of sense". If an idea
or an image were only thought by one mind, its apprehension by
another clearly involves Telepathy.

It is also not clairvoyance, which means a power to see
what is hidden from ordinary physical sight. We are living all
the while surrounded by a vast ocean of mingled air and
electromagnetic waves, the latter inter-penetrating the former,
as it does all physical matter; and it is chiefly by means of
vibrations in that vast ocean of energy that impressions reach
us from the outside. Clairvoyance like many other things in
nature is mainly a question of vibrations and is in fact nothing
but an extension of powers which we are all using every day in
our lives.

In Telepathy "symbolism" of idea, sound, feeling, emotion
etc. plays an important role in the mechanism of transmission;
where as in clairvoyance the image of the visual or auditory
reality is itself the object of transmission and no interpretation
of that image is necessary. If radiation and vibration were
involved in Telepathy, radiation of thought is observed but in
clairvoyance the perception of radiation is objective reality.

No doubt, Telepathy also plays a great role in curing
diseases. The patients at distant place are influenced by
thought waves or vibrations of saints or experts in this art
without administering any drug. The raised emotionalism of
the sender releases his radiating power and turns a latent
faculty to radiate into an actual and powerful radiation.

Effects of transmission of drug-energy through detached
hair of the patient cannot be called "Telepathy as it is so simple.
No exercise of mind or effort is done on the part of the
transmitter. Select a right remedy for a patient and hand it over

to even a lay man with instructions, he can very easily transmit by bringing it in contact with a hair of the patient. Emphatically it can be ascertained that transmission of drug-energy has nothing to do with Telepathy or clairvoyance.

4.   Is It Spirit Healing ?

There are some people who use to say that there is some spiritual power in the author's hand or it is spirit healing. The spirit healing is healing from spirit, through spirit, to the spirit-body of he patient and thence to the physical body of the patient. The healing vibrations that are used in spirit healing are of divine source coming direct from God. They are precisely the same vibrations as used by Jesus Christ the Great Healer that ever lived and later by his disciples in the performance of healing miracles. Spirit healing is prevalent in England and other countries. There is a great healing centre at Birminghum where the sick from various parts of the country are treated. Dr. W. Lang, F.R.C.S., an Ophthalmic surgeon of London, of a great acumen died on 13.7.1937. George Chapman of Aylesbury Fire Brigade is the medium of the Late Dr. Lang, who has performed operations on the spirit body of hundreds of patients. Even at a distance the patients have been cured by him through his medium. J. Bernard Hutton says in his book, "HEALING HANDS" that leukemia, kidney stones, paralysis, spondylitis, cancer, blindness etc. have been cured. He himself has got his lost sight back through the medium of Chapman.

Dr. E.T. Baily, M.B.B.S., F.R.C.S. has narrated in the introduction of this book that it is the true story of "Miracles" wrought by spirit healing through the devoted medium, George Chapman and the late famous surgeon Dr. William Lang.

Transmission of drug-energy is neither the spirit healing as people call nor the author is a medium of any spirit.

5.   Evolution of Theory Involved in
Drug Transmission.

If the effect of drug transmission on the patient through his hair separated from his body is neither psychological nor Telepathic etc. then what is the rationale behind it? The author tried his level best to find it out and how the theory was evolved gradually is given below.

In the beginning of his discovery, the phenomenon was explained by citing examples of scorpion or Snake-bites and

Alsatian dog which run like this. When a scorpion bites a person, it is not killed, rather its movement is restricted by covering it with a small basket. It is said that if the scorpion moves fast, the person bitten has intense burning pain and if it moves slowly intensity of pain is less, and if it sits without any motion, intensity is very-very less. This shows the relationship between the scorpion and its poison even after its separation from it. In the same way the hair has got relation with the body even after its separation and any energy applied to it (hair) is transmitted to the person concerned through invisible trail left by the hair. Similarly when a snake bites a person, the snake is not allowed to be killed. This belief is prevalent in the rural areas since long. Why so? Perhaps it is believed that when the snake is alive, there is a chance of taking the poison injected into the body back and the victim may be saved, but if it is killed, poison will remain in his body and he is bound to die. It may mean that there is invisible relation between the injected poison and the snake at a distance. In the same way when hair is detached from the body there is relationship between the hair and the person; and if any subtle energy (drug) is brought in contact with that hair, the person is affected by it at a distance.

Similarly the example of Alsatian dog was cited to explain the phenomenon. When burglary is committed, Alsatian dog is brought to the site of offence. The Culprit leaves behind him a trail of smell connecting him with that site. The sense of smell of the A. dog is very acute and it can detect the invisible trail of smell left behind by the culprit. The dog through that trail of smell of the culprit's belonging goes from the site to him (Culprit). In the same way when a hair is detached from the patient's body and is brought to the doctor, there is an invisible trail left behind by the hair from the patient to the doctor and thus both are connected by the trail, and when dynamic drug is brought in contact with the hair, its energy is transmitted along that invisible trail to the patient and thus the medicinal energy affects him at a distance. These analogies do not seem correct and appealing hence another field was hunted out. An attempt was made to offer a scientific explanation of the process of transmission of Homoeo drug energy with the help of an idea of "IONISATION" in the following way.

"The human body is composed of cells consisting of innumerable atoms and there is a network of nerve-wires for receiving and transmitting impulses. The Bell Telephone Laboratory of New York City has discovered that human body is radiating energy at the rate of 80 million cycles per second. The body which is itself a store-house of energy, always emanates and receives energy in the shape of electro-magnetic waves. The Electric Encephalograph demonstrates today the radiation of electro-magnetic waves from the brain of human body. The vital force in the body is the electrical equilibrium of all the vibrations, radiations and reception of different cells constituting the body and any disturbance in this equilibrium gives room to a disease".

"The crude drug is divided and subdivided by attenuations into electrically charged particles called Ions. Hence the potentised drug is nothing but energy in ionised form, which forms an electrical field in the phial. When this potentised drug is put on the tongue, it gets charged and activised by the nerve of the tongue which is already electrically charged. This is how Homoeopathic drug acts through the oral method".

"In the case of transmission of drug rather its curative energy through the medium of a separated hair of a patient, the same electrical equilibrium of the body is affected by the field of the drug. Modern Forensic Science has proved that though two faces may be similar in appearance, the striations of fingers and hairs of one individual differ from those of other individual and these striations and hair may have a specific relation with the body of that particular individual. The hair of a particular man represents the same constitution in a miniature form, of which the particular man is himself made of. The hair has got the same characteristic vibration as that of the body of the individual and this capacity of vibration, capacity to receive and transmit energy of a particular quality is unchanged, even after the hair or any part of the body is detached or separated from the body, provided of course the physical form of the detached portion is not changed. As in the case of a body, the hair also is electrically charged. The potentised drug remains in its ionised form in a polarized state having its own electrical field. And when this field comes in contact with the field of the hair, the resultant field becomes so intense and rapid that it begins to radiate energy, waves or pulses at a particular frequency. As the constitution and vibratory state of hair, which transmits the resultant energy (effect of medicine) is the same as that of the body from which the hair was detached (patient), this vibration of hair caused by the effect of medicine causes a similar and sympathetic vibration in the body, i.e. the reservoir of the electrical energy of the patient, affecting the patient in the same way, as the drug energy acts when put on the tongue. The propagation of vibration of the effect or drug does not require actual physical contact of drug with body as it is only the energy of drug which is transmitted in a similar way as that of Radio and Television".

The above explanation is not so sound because the theory of IONISATION may not be equally applicable in case of all the Homoeopathic drugs obtained from various sources. Efforts were made to find out the general explanation and ultimately a new idea of transmission based on emission of electromagnetic waves and *"Raman Effect"* has been developed which has been discussed in detail in Chapter VI under the caption "Mechanism of drug transmission", in part II of this book. Now the discovery has got scientific as well as experimental supports.

CHAPTER II
THE HUMAN ORGANISM
AN ELECTRICAL SYSTEM

If the gross like sound and light can be transmitted then why not the subtle energy of Homoeo medicines. Let us now find out the distinction between the gross and the subtle. The gross are those which can be sensed by the sensory organs like nose, ears, eyes, tongue and skin. Smell is sensed by the olfactory organ, (nose), sound by auditory organs (ears), sight by visual organs (eyes), taste by gustatory organ (tongue) and touch by tactual organ (skin). Hence smell, sound etc. are gross.

The subtle are those which cannot be sensed by these external organs of knowledge. The spirit or soul is subtle. Internal organ is needed to perceive its subtle nature. Mind is not made of the material elements (bhutas) like the external senses. It is not limited to the knowledge of any particular class of things or qualities, but functions as a central co-ordinating organ in all kinds of knowledge. It is an internal sense. The energy liberated in the potentised medicine is just like soul in the body and hence it is subtle.

Now let us come to the physical science for its explanation as to how the Homoeo. drug-energy acts through the uprooted hair of the patient. For the purpose of discussion the subject is divided into the following :—

(1) The human organism-an electrical system.
(2) The vital Principle.
(3) Disease.
(4) The drug and potency.
(5) The Mechanism of Drug Transmission.

In this chapter only "The human oganism—an electrical system" is discussed, the rest of the subject will be discussed in subsequent Chapters.

The Human Organism—An Electrical System.

The whole universe is an effect of some cause, the material as well as efficient. The efficient cause is not our subject here as it concerns Metaphysics. The universe is composed of elements, molecules and atoms. The human body is composed of many cells and tissues, which too are made of molecules and atoms. The organism is an electrically charged living machine. It resembles spontaneously. The whole administration is managed by the mind. There is a systematic network of communication called nervous system. There are approximately ten billion neurons in the human brain only. Each neuron contains an electrical charge and each cell is a fully charged small battery. The nervous system is a most complicated and highly organised body. The nerve tissue consists of nerve cells and nerve fibres. This system may be divided into two subdivisions — the cerebro-spinal and the automatic. The cerebro-spinal system is composed of a central and a peripheral part. The central part consists of the brain and medulla spinalis or spinal cord. These two parts constitute the central nervous system.

Dr. S. Close, M.D. Says, "The Central nervous system may be compared to a dynamo. As a dynamo is a machine, driven by steam or some other force, which, through the agency of electromagnetic induction from a surrounding magnetic field, converts into electrical energy in the form of current the mechanical energy expended upon it, so the central nervous system is a machine driven by chemical force derived from food, through the agency of electro-vital induction from a surrounding vital field, converts into vital energy, in the form of nerve current or impulses, the chemo-physical energy expended upon it."

Further he says, "As an electrical transportation system depends for its working force upon the dynamo located in its central station, so the human body depends for the force necessary to carry on its operation upon the central power station, located in the central nervous system".

The automatic system again consists of (i) efferent fibres (motor nerves) to convey electric currents or impulses from the central nervous system—the headquarter to the other parts, and (ii) afferent fibres (sensory nerves) to transmit impulses or electric currents from other parts to the brain. Take for example a prick in the finger and see how it acts. As soon as the finger is pricked the impulse (electric current) is transmitted through the afferent nerve to brain and order comes from the centre through the efferent fibres giving an electrical shock (jerk) to take the hand off the site of trouble and thus the equilibrium is maintained. Two-way traffic works here. This process takes place automatically in no time. Dr. Bellokossy Says, "It is evident that such a rapid Communication of messages to all the regions of the body, adjacent and remote & this general engagement of the cell's defenses through the nervous channels cannot possibly be of chemical nature. It can only be by electrical induction & reflex actions which spreads from cell to cell with lightning speed".

Glifforo, C. Furnas in his book "Next Hundred Years" has stated that an adult human body consists of 1000,000,000,000,000,000 cells. These cells are produced from one cell-fertilized ovum. These are a complex of protein molecules which contain mainly Carbon, Oxygen, Hydrogen, Nitrogen, Phosphorus and Sulphur. Each cell is produced from electric unit or wave packet. In this way it can be said that the human body is a complex of 1.8×10^{28} wave packets.

The Bell Telephone Laboratories of New York City has discovered that human bodies radiate or vibrate. The rate of radiation is eighty million cycles per second, but the rate of electrical energy which produces ordinary light is only sixty cycles. That is why the radiations of our bodies are not perceived by our eyes. Dr. Morton Whitley in his book "Theory of Life, Disease and Death" states that life exists only because of electrical energy of living matter which is the sum total of collective tissue energy. In the inorganic matter it is dynamic. In the human body there is always a flow of electric waves in the nervous system. According to Dr. Harold S. Buw of Yak University, every living thing is a storage of battery charged with energy we call electricity. The electric waves emanating from the brain are graphed by the powerful instrument called Cathode Ray Oscillograph.

How human radiations can be used in curing diseases may be read in "Co-operative Healing—The Curative Properties of Human Radiations" by Mr. L.E. Eman. Mr. E. Eman has cured various ailments by human radiations by a circuit linking positives with negatives. All human beings are electro-magnetically positive at head, right hand and foot and negative at the base of spine, left hand and foot. The conducted wireless radiations emitted by the human body can be used therapeutically, provided that Polar opposites are linked by electrical conductors. Mr. E. Eman used insulated copper wire and copper gauze mats to link the opposite poles—positive and negative in one body or several bodies. Any circuit linking positives with negatives is beneficial to health, and any reversal of it is harmful. Any arrangement which connects polar opposites or of different bodies by means of electrical conductors is referred to as a "relaxation circuit" and any arrangement which connects polar similars as a "tension circuit". The relaxation circuit automatically promotes relaxation of the voluntary muscles and stimulates the functional activity. It fosters sleep, recovery from fatigue and disease. Capacity for work and health in general, while the tension circuit waves reverse the effects. Both circuits affect not only organic but also nervous and mental health.

The scientists regard the earth as a huge natural magnet. All living organisms-the human, animals and plants, and the inanimate objects receive magnetic energy transmitted from the earth. The man takes full advantage of the magnetic energy in a varied way, along with other organisms. Birds enjoy a change of place thousands of miles away across the sea, solely being guided by their instincts to fly along the magnetic lines of the earth.

Our body also is a small natural magnet. The head and upper half of the body represent the North Pole and the lower half of the body and feet represent the South Pole. Atoms, the minutest constituents of the body are manifestations of electrons, protons, and other particles, full of electric energy, which sustains life. Its presence in the body is life, and its absence is death.

The whole universe is balanced by magnetism, and so is the man. The magnetic force is greatly manifested through mind and spiritual tendencies of man, which may vary in intensity and effect. Magnetic energy provides immense power to mind and body to perform wonders and miracles. Great ones, having intense magnetic power, invisibly guide the millions to their destination. A magnetic personality has the power to attract others towards him or to prevail upon other's mind.

Man's mind is regulated by magnetic force which is responsible for his happiness, joys, laughter, delights, smile etc. on the one hand and griefs, sorrows, melancholy, desponding, lamentations, fear etc. on the other.

As we know iron is sensitive to magnet. In human body haemoglobin in blood attracts magnetic forces and provides the cells with electric energy to carry on their functions properly. Any decrease in the intake of this energy causes sickness and absence of it leads to death. Obviously, development of physical health and advancement of mental faculty depend entirely on the magnetic forces. A good health and happy life indicates an optimum presence of electric forces in the body whereas lack of it is manifested in ill health and unhappy life. In good health cells and tissues of the body are charged with sparking electric waves, in absence of which cells die and bacteria finds a place to develop and proliferate.

This magnetic power was well known to our ancient Rishis who demonstrated this in performing wonders and miracles. The Hindu scriptures also lay down the principles regulating an ideal life of man, some of which are highly scientific. For example, stretching the body North-South in sleep, so as to place the head towards the North, is regarded as beneficial to sound sleep.

Our body, though it looks small, has a vast potential magnetic power in it. Unless we recognize it and feel it within ourselves, we shall have to depend on energy from outside. This is possible only through scientific meditation. But this is not possible for all. Therefore, care has to be taken to conserve this energy in the body by allowing more energy to get in through regulating our habits of eating, sleeping and working. A moderate yogic exercise is helpful.

The magnetic energy has been and is being put to various uses in the world. Wide Claims have been made in the field of medical Service in curing the functional defects of the body. Some incurable cases are also reported to have been cured.

Every object of the universe gives off radiation, hence human beings are not an exception. The halo of Aura of this radiations has been shown around the head of God, Goddess or saints like Ram, Krishna, Mahavir, Budha, Christ etc. in religious literatures. This aura is not confined to the saint alone. Every object has this. In Russia & the U.S.A. the photograph of this aura radiating from leaves or human beings etc. has been taken successfully. This will be shown in details in the next chapter. This is called bioplasma or electromagnetic field of the person or object photographed.

There are many examples of persons having electrical charges which would be easily felt like electric currents. A circular galaxy was observed for a few seconds around the chest of a lady named Anna Monari in the hospital of Pirani in Italy in 1934. This galaxy was observed for weeks together when she was fast asleep covered with sweat. Rapid respirations and palpitations of heart were also seen. The news spread like wildfire & scientists,—Biologists, Physicists, Physicians press reporters from all over the world rushed there to see that miracle. Dr. K. Sage opined that the phenomenon took place due to electromagnetic induction. Another scientist opined that electromagnetic radiations induced due to certain chemical reactions in the skin was the cause of that phenomenon. There are certain examples of electrical shocks by the human electricity. Miss. J. Smith of Ireland had a such huge amount of electricity in her body that it would give shocks on touching her body. Under the leadership of Dr. S. Kapt, it was examined & found out true. Suddenly electrical currents began to flow in the body of a girl named Jeni Morgan aged 14 of Missoui Sidalia village near Berlin (Germany). Her body was behaving just like powerful battery. One day, while she was pulling water by hand pump, sparks of fire began to come out from the place, she held the handle of the pump. She got afraid & narrated this incidence to her family members. First it was thought that electric currents might have come in the pump from any source but on examination & test it was not found true, rather the girl's body was full of electrical energy. Whomsoever, she could touch, he or she felt electrical shocks. In this way she had been untouched for many years & in due course it gradually disappeared.

It is the effect of human electricity that one attracts or influences the other. Beauty is the manifestation of this energy The blooming youth becomes the centre of attractions. If this human electricity is preserved it can be utilized for useful purposes. By channelising this energy into multifaced genius, brilliance & power, many miraculous & important achievements can be made. Thus Brahman, warriors, saints, philosophers, scientists, leaders and the genius in other fields have tasted the nectar of this energy. Sometimes it comes to a certain person automatically. This can be developed by yogic practices. The human organism endowed with the vital energy is a very very sensitive living Radioset. It receives energies from the cosmic source through innumerable pores and hairs. It also emanates through them. The hair, a part of the body has the same or similar vibrations or characteristics as that of the body. It is amphoteric in nature. Hairs serve as antennas for the human organism.

CHAPTER III

VITAL PRINCIPLE

Medical science in its infancy was just a part of other sciences and for a long time it was monopolised by the priests, saints and philosophers. Medical science has all the time been influenced by the philosophical thoughts in the country. During the days of Hahnemann there were three schools of philosophy- materialism, idealism and transcendentalism. According to materialism the real world is that which is visible and explained. Idealism is "that system of reflective thinking which would interpret and explain the whole universe, things and minds and their relations, as the realization of a system of ideas. It takes various forms as determined by the view of what the idea or the ideal is, and of how we become aware of it." Transcendentalism shares the ideas of both the doctrines and pleads something above these two. Lord Bacon has compared the first with ants which know nothing except collecting and hoarding things; the second the spider which goes on spinning cob-webs and the third with the honey-bee which collects raw materials from outside world and manufactures honey. Hahnemann was very much influenced by the latter. For the practical purposes he adopted the Lord Bacon's inductive logic. He was unprejudiced observer and he accepted the facts as he found them. To him matter, force, energy, motion, body, mind, soul, consciousness and super-consciousness, all were realities. For him the human body is a divine creation having 'dynamis' or 'life force'.

As already stated in the earlier chapter, the human body is an automatic machinery and it functions like an electric system. The functions of different organs of the body are regulated by different controlling centres to the brain through a network of nerves. Now the question arises as to what is that which makes this complicated machinery run smoothly and uninterruptedly? How is its existence possible? Naturally it comes to mind that there must be a system of unalterable relations, perpetuated by some single unifying principle. One organ of the body has definite relations with the other organs and the units-cells working harmoniously presuppose the existence of a vital principle which itself is a part thereof. Obviously, something that establishes harmonious relations in the functioning of this body cannot be a constituent element. There must be some principle working behind all this and this is vital principle.

According to the experiences of the Indian Saints 'Man' is encircled by the seven forms of bodies—(1) Physical body, (2) etheric body, (3) astral body, (4) mental body, (5) spiritual body, (6) cosmic body and (7) bodyless body. The last one can only be attained after liberation (Moksh).

The vital principle is a conscious substance having consciousness as its attributes. It is a propelling energy to manoeuvre the living machine from within. It is a life-principle by virtue of which all the organisms evolve and with its exhaustion and extinction, they decay. It is a like a sum total of electric energy in the body which flows in every cell through the nervous system and maintains the equilibrium. Hahnemann regarded the vital principle as unintelligible whereas Kent viewed it as intelligible. According to Hahnemann "In the healthy force (autocracy) the dynamis that animates the material body (organism) rules with unbounded sway, and retains all the parts of the organism in admirable, harmonious vital operation, as regards both sensations and functions, so that our indwelling reason gifted mind can freely employ this living, healthy instrument for the higher purposes of our existence". In this statement Dr. Hahnemann, the father of Homoeopathy, leaves the ground and flies in the metaphysical world. Further he states in Section 10 of the Organon that the material organism, without the vital force, is capable of no sensations, no function, no self-preservation, it derives all sensations and performs all functions of life solely by means of the immaterial being (the vital force-the vital principle) which animates the material organism in health and disease. The vital principle animates the body and keeps it in healthy condition. In the universe everything has some purpose and has its own beginning and end. So is the case with man. He has certain purposes and after fulfillment of these he passes away. But from the beginning to the end there is a continuous link or chain, one linking the other without any breakage. This continuity is maintained by the vital principle.

The vital principle is subject to changes. It may be in order or disorder in varying degrees. It is influenced by external as well as internal forces. The man himself is a powerful agent to bring about changes in vital principle. Vital principle pervades the entire material body without disturbing or replacing it and it also dominates and controls it. Our body exhibits a wonderful co-ordination and harmony which is maintained by vital principle, without which the material body is dead.

Its quality can be predicted only in degrees. It adapts itself to the surroundings and thus keeps the human body in order under all circumstances. It keeps the human body continuously constructed and when it is withdrawn from a particular part of the body or from the body as a whole, the different forces in the body are controlled by the vital principle and total absence of control results in decay or death of the body. It not only controls the human body as a whole, it also controls the units in the same way. If we examine the plasma body, we find that it has all the essentials of life that the highest order of life has. It reproduces itself, activates itself, propagates and finally dies. After death everything is there in the body and there is no decrease in the weight of the body but what is that which kept it alive. The chemical analysis cannot justify it, as all this is related to a phenomenon of electrical or spirit like energy.

This vital principle not only pervades and illuminates the body but also sends out radiations in the shape of halo or aura. This aura has been depicted, in our ancient literature, around the bodies of saints, with golden halos around the heads. The scientists have been trying to find out means to make this phenomenon visible.

This emanation or emission has been variously described as 'corona discharge', 'bioplasma body', 'aura', etc. Cold emissions of electrons have been described by Americans as 'corona discharge'; 'bioplasma body' is descriptive of the emanations and internal structure of the objects photographed, and 'aura' is subtle emanations.

This aura is present not only around the Saints' heads but all things in the universe have their own atmosphere (aura)—

the Sun, the Moon, the planets, the stars, etc. Every living being also has its own aura or atmosphere.

These radiations or subtle emanations have been photographed by a method of producing photographs from the action of high frequency currents. This is known as Kirlian photography. This is able to show the man's experiments with the forces inside and outside the body.

Green leaves and dried leaves have been photographed which show variations in emanations. Photography of the various stages in the death of a leaf showed withdrawal of radiation from the atmosphere, and with the life force moving inwards there was a change in colour of the leaf.

In a laboratory some 500 persons were photographed which revealed that each one revealed in his corona a distinct pattern from every other man. In photography of fingers, no two fingers could be found to have the same aura. Even the same finger photographed after a day showed changes in corona discharge. A photograph taken of a man in normal condition and the other taken after he got drunk showed that alcohol clearly changed the corona, which in the latter case was sketchy, suggestive of nervousness or anxiety.

Researches have been conducted to examine the psychological state under the influence of drugs, hypnosis, meditation, yogic exercises, etc. and varying degrees of changes in the corona discharge have been found in each case. In a normal condition a small red blotch was seen while in self induced trance, the corona was blue-white.

Yogic breathing exercises and meditation increase the size of corona. In the relaxed condition the corona was brilliant and wider, whereas in tension and emotional excitement red bloches were found. Size of corona was also found to be influenced by the change of photographers, from one person to another or from a male to a female or from an unknown to a known photographer. In case of a female and a friend photographer corona was brighter. Experiment showed that blue and white colours are prominent in subjects who are in the higher realm of consciousness, beyond alpha and past theta, and practising transcendental meditation.

Radiation field photography reveals a highly complex and unknown phenomenon. It is related to invisible energy system which has also been described in ancient Indian text, such as Bhagvat Gita.

The vital principle has been referred to,in the Hindu scrip tures as 'Prana'. It is vital or cosmic energy which sustains and regulates the whole body. Prana is life of all living organisms. It has the power of regeneration and rejuvenation. It is a creative "lifetronic" forces, beyond the atom, and finer electronic energy.

The body-battery of man is sustained by vibratory cosmic energy or (Aum) and the invisible powers flow into the body through the medula oblongata, the sixth spinal chakra.

The Bible refers to Prana as invisible life force or as Holy ghost that upholds all creations.

This life energy or Prana lies dormant, unawakened and unused, in Kundalini. Therefore, though this body looks small, it has immense power in it. This power is intrinsically linked with the physical or mental body. This power (super Pran-shakti) can be awakened by Yoga. By Yoga this can be controlled and distributed to all parts of the body equally, or it may be withdrawn to a particular part. Prana, when awakened by Yoga, fills the body with electrical energy. This life energy or Prana is subject to modification, amplification and transformation to varied degrees. To arouse this power one has to go through a specific technique and regular practice of yogic kriya. Thus, when Prana is controlled, it is possible to send it to a particular part of the body where its presence may be required for the purposes of healing or otherwise. Miraculous healing can be affected by control of Prana and its distribution in the body.

Prana is the body of the self (Supreme consciousness). It is the vehicle or medium of consciousness. In this sense Prana can be equated with the Indian concept of prakriti, which means the manifested constituents of the universe in the form of matter and energy. This Prana is energy for carrying conscious-ness. Without Prana, consciousness would be totally unable to express itself in the Phenomenal world to manifest the myriads of life-forms in the Universe. Prana is the active aspect of existence and consciousness is the all pervading, inactive and witnessing principle. For life to exist, both must be present.

In ancient China the concept of universal energy was

prevalent. Instead of Prana they call it "Ki". The universal energy is constituted of two continually and mutually interacting principles called "Yin and Yang". The manifested universe is seen a harmonious whole and subject to change through the ceaseless interplay of the complimentary and eternally changing Yin and Yang. Yin and Yang can be considered as the negative and positive forces, the two poles of the manifested whole. The two aspects Yin and Yang are interdependent and interlocking parts of the whole, each containing within itself, the germ of potential of the other. These principles are encompassed or held together by the "Tao-Consciousness".

The modern science has also postulated that the basic substance of the infinite cosmos around us in energy. In this respect science, Yoga and other ancient systems have agreed with each other. The physical body is evolved and controlled by the Pranic body.

Electromagnetic Phenomena play a vital role in the ecology of consciousness. Magnetic and particularly electromagnetic fields have enormous implications for understanding of consciousness. All objects in the Universe with a temperature above absolute zero emit electromagnetic radiation. According to the pioneers of electromagnetic theory of life—Prof. S. Burr, Prof. of Anatomy at Yale University and Leonard J. Ravitz a Psychiatrist-electromagnetic fields guide the growth and repair of living protoplasm. This discovery of the field they called the Life-field.

Prof. Burr states that if we meet a friend after six months, there is not one molecule in his face that was there when we saw him. There is a constant turnover of the materials in our bodies and brains; all the protein is renewed every six months. How do we recognize our friend after six months if he has changed so much? Burr says that it is the Life-field which controls it.

According to the Indian ancient saints, Yogis and Seers ten pranas function as just this type of organizational matrix. It is a good way to understand the functions of Prana in the body. We have to know the man who is a multidimensional being and has unlimited consciousness. His consciousness can be measured through its effects. It is capable of expansion and it has been photographed. The Psychic Phenomena are no longer a matter of speculation, they are proven, well documented facts.

Every man receives as well as transmits electromagnetic energy in the form of waves. We are not separate from the rest of the universe but a part of everything that lives and has its being. The PRANA or vital principle, maintaining, developing, repairing, sustaining and illuminating the whole organism projects itself outside the body also in the shape of "electrobio-luminescence", aura, "bioplasma" or electromagnetic field around the body which has capacity to influence others and receive radiations from different sources.

CHAPTER IV

DISEASE

Disease is just a departure of the human organism from its normal conditions that constitute health and, therefore, it will be appropriate here to say first something about health.

Health is a condition of body in which the vital principle animates the organism and keeps the body in harmonious order. In health the body is charged with electric energy and is capable of normal sensations, self-preservation and performing normal functions. Above all, it keeps the body and mind in perfect order so that these might work ceaselessly towards the attainment of the goal of life.

Plainly speaking health is taken to mean a natural condition of the body which is free from any disease. Sound development of body and mind, resistance to disease and harmonious functioning of the different organs of the body constitute health. Thus the term 'health' presupposes four factors : sound body, sound mind, healthy morals and vital strength. Here we have to take into consideration the fact that in Homoeopathy besides the above four, the spiritual health is all the more important.

The term 'disease' is very controversial in Homoeopathy. In Organon more emphasis has been laid on 'sickness' than on 'disease'. The reason is that sickness is prior to disease. It will, therefore, be proper here to throw some light on sickness also. The very first Section of Organon reads as follows — "The physician's high and only mission is to restore the sick to health, to cure, as it is termed". It is the man who is sick, and not his organs. In some cases we come across patients who complain of so many troubles and report that there is nothing wrong with them as they have gone in for all the pathological tests. But the fact that troubles are there with them is enough to corroborate that they are sick. If this sickness is allowed to continue uncured, after lapse of certain period, organs will be affected and the body will be diseased. The fact is that the organs which are giving out various sensations are just manifesting the internal disorders.

Now the question arises what constitutes man ? According to Hahnemann, "Combination of the will and the understanding constitute man; conjoined they make life and activity, they manufacture the body and cause all things of the body....The man is will and understanding and the house which he lives in is his body". The maintenance of this body depends on correct thinking and understanding and deviation from the order is bound to cause damage to the body.

But in this world man is more materialist than spiritualist. Naturally his life on earth is a mixture of joys and sorrows. Even if it be possible for him to avoid pains and miseries, it is impossible to evade the clutches of decay and death. It is said that the body is the abode of diseases. All the living beings, being effects of some cause undergo changes, decay and death, hence man also is not free from this universal law. This world is a moral stage for education and emancipations. Ordinarily he is the victim of three kinds of diseases, i.e. the Adhyatamika, Adhibhautika and Adhidaivika. The first is due to intra-organic causes like bodily disorders and mental afflictions. It includes both bodily and mental diseases, such as Rheumatism, Cancer, Fever, Headache, pangs of fear, anger, blast etc. The second is caused by the extra-organic natural causes, like enemy, beasts, poisonous insects. The third is produced by the extra-organic supernatural causes like pains inflicted by demons, ghosts, etc. The vital principle of Dr. S. Hahnemann is enjoyer and sufferer unlike the soul of the Sankhya and the Vedanta philosophy for which it is pure consciousness and Satchittanand-existence-consciousness-bliss respectively. The body, of course, is a material instrument of life. In the Organon in section 11 and 12, it is stated that when a person falls ill, it is only this spiritual self acting (automatic) vital principle, everywhere present in his organism, that is primarily deranged by the dynamic influence upon it of a morbific agent inimical to life; it is only the vital principle, deranged to such an abnormal state, that can furnish the organism with its disagreeable sensations and incline it to the irregular processes which we call disease; for, as powerful and invisible in itself and only cognizable by its effects on the organism, its morbid derangement only makes itself known by the manifestation of disease in the sensations and functions of those parts of the organism exposed to the senses of the observer and physician, that is, by morbid symptoms, and in no other way can make itself known.

"It is morbidly affected vital force alone that produces diseases, so that the morbid phenomena perceptible to our senses express at the same time all the internal change, that is to say, the whole morbid derangement of the internal dynmic in a word, they reveal the whole disease, consequently, also the disappearance under treatment of all the morbid phenomena of all the morbid alterations that differ from the healthy vital operations, certainly affects and necessarily implies the restoration of the integrity of the vital force and, therefore, the recovered health of the whole organism".

Our vital principle is a spirit-like dynamic and it is affected also in a spirit-like dynamic way (Disease) and is cured by the spirit-like dynamic way (medicine). The diseases are nothing more than alterations in the state of health. The flow of energy is disturbed by the dynamic morbid agent. The equilibrium of health is disturbed. The vital principle is dynamic and disease is also dynamic. The disease is nothing but the counter-current force on the vital principle hence there is a chaos or conflict in the organism and sign and symptoms are the call of the vital principle. The affection of the vital principle and the diseased one are the same.

Now it is clear that the disease is the result of the altered functioning of the vital principle.. Its causations are (a) exciting causes—influence of emotion, atmosphere, micro-organism, poison, drugs, etc.—producing acute disease; mild or fatal; (b) contributory causes—that which contributes to the perpetuation of a condition, such as damp places, unhygienic working condition, etc.; and (c) miasmatic causes—psora, syphilis and sycosis. These are responsible for both (a) acute diseases—epidemic, sporadic, personal etc. and (b) chronic diseases caused by psora, syphilis and sycosis. Their first effect is seen in the changes in the cells. In this condition there is no visible change. Slowly and secretly the disease force goes deeper and deeper and its effects travel from finer to coarser and coarser to outermost man when sensations of varying degrees are felt.

Psora is the mother of all diseases. Hahnemann refers to psora as the oldest and universal chronic miasmatic disease. It is psora which prepares the ground for development of the two other miasms, syphilis and sycosis. It is the first and primary disorder of the human being. It found its birth with the very primitive wrong of the human race with its spiritual sickness. This spiritual sickness progressed with the human race and came to be known as susceptibility laying down foundation for diseases of various kinds. Generation after generation it grew stronger and stronger and with the villainous influence of drugs, which always tried to suppress it and drive it inside and make it invisible, it developed into a powerful invisible enemy of human race. Today it is the most infectious of all the chronic diseases. The fact is that its outer manifestations in the form of itch and eruptions on skin have all the time been suppressed and driven inside. Its suppression causes diseases like tuberculosis, asthma, gout, epilepsy, ulcer, cancer, haemorhoids, insanity, etc.

The other two chronic miasms have venerial origin. Syphilis has three stages—primary,secondary and tertiary. After the later stage it produces nervous symptoms, mental symptoms and cardiovascular symptoms. Sycosis in the first stage is known by gonorrhea, in the second by venereal warts or sycotic condylomata over the genitals and in the third, when it has been suppressed, it attacks heart, mind, bone, etc.

The human body takes a miasm only once in his life time and this goes with him till the end of his life unless it is eradicated by proper remedy. Psora with the other miasms produces complex diseases, difficult to get rid of. These miasms may remain in the body until circumstances awaken it. These are transmitted from generation to generation through genes manifestations of which are seen in varying degrees.

Now let us see what effects do the diseases have on the radiation of vital principle. As already said in the previous chapter, the emanations of vital principle are subject to change in accordance with the physical, mental and psychological condition of the man. In diseased condition the emissions in regard to both, wavelength and brilliance, have been found to be quite different from those found in the normal condition. Simoneton found that the normal healthy person gives off a radiation of about '6500 angstroms' or a little higher, whereas the radiations given off by tobacco smokers, alcohol imbibers and carrion eaters are uniformly lower. Bovis claimed that cancer patients gives off a wavelength of '4875 angstroms'.

Thus, we see that the radiation has definite relation with the physical and mental conditions. Not only this, the physical or mental condition of man is also affected by radiations of other entities. A healthy man living with the T.B. or cancer patients may be affected by the radiations coming out of these patients. All this phenomenon has in the back ground a constant interaction of energies. In the words of Bellokossy "Life is interaction of energies which are propagated indefinitely in induction. Homoeopathy deals with life by means of energy in the form of potencies produced by interaction".

CHAPTER V

THE DRUG AND POTENCY

Life in the world is full of sufferings. There is its cause. It is possible to get rid of it and there is path which leads to the cessation of it. The attempt to put an end to suffering gave birth to the medical science and other measures—Telepathy, Mantras, Ojha, Spirit healing etc. from time to time according to the advancement of civilization. The earth is full of medicinal substances and they are utilised for the purpose according to the respective medical principles. Dr. S. Hahnemann was born at a time when there was a great upsurge of different philosophical and scientific thoughts and were educated in the modern school of medicine. He was a lover of truth and he saw the defects in that school which is based on the principle of "Contraria Contraris" and discovered the right path to cure disease gently, rapidly and permanently by giving the world, the immortal principle of "Similia Similibus Curenter". The like are cured by the like. The principle is not a new phenomenon for India. "Vishashya Visha Aushadham" is an old principle in our ancient literature which means that poison neutralises the effect of poison. The same substance may be used by different Schools of medicines but the approach is quite different from one another. It may be used on the "Contraria Contrary" or the "Similia Similibus Curenter" principles. There are different sources of drugs. They are (1) The mineral kingdom—Gold, Silver, (2) The vegetable kingdom—Aloe, Lycopodium, (3) The animal kingdom—Apis, Lachesis, (4) The nosodes-derived from disease-products—Tuberculinum, (5) The sarcodes-remedies prepared from the healthy tissue and secretions—Thyroidinum, (6) The imponderabilia—Radium, X-Ray etc. Each and every drug has its own potentiality and its action differs from that of every other. Only that substance is called drug or medicine which has capacity to produce and cure disease. Every substance has indwelling curative power which is disease-producing as well as the disease-curing power and this power is spirit-like. Dr. S. Hahnemann states that this spirit-like power to alter man's state of health(and hence to cure diseases) which lies hidden in the inner nature of medicines, can never be discovered by us by a mere effort of reason, it is only by experience of the phenomena it displays when acting on the state of health of man that we can become clearly cognizant of it. This curative principle in medicines is not in itself percep- tible. This principle is energy and can be arrived at by certain processes, which lead to Dynamisation theory of drugs.

The crude medicinal substances reveal their medicinal power by the process of triturations or succussion. It is done by dilution and friction. The Homoeopathic dynamisations are the real awakenings of the medicinal properties hidden in the crude substance. This is done by dividing and sub-dividing the crude medicinal substance by dilution. As for example, one drop of the tincture is mixed with 99 drops of alcohol and given succussions to make 1st potency. Now one drop from 1st potency mixed with 99 drops of fresh alcohol gives 2nd potency and so on. It means that the 1st potency contains 10^{-2} part of the original medicine and the 2nd potency contains 10^{-4} only. In the 12th or in some case 15th potency we reach the stage of atom which is 10^{-24} or 10^{-30}. Still we go higher and higher by dividing and sub-dividing.

Practically the more we decrease the quantity of a drug, the more powerful it becomes. Why it is so, it is still a question ? A number of views has been expressed to account for the enhanced reactivity of Homoeopathic drugs with rise of potency. A few of them may be mentioned here.

(1)   Idea of Ionisation :Taking help of idea of ionisation many thinkers say that when electrolytes undergo ionisation and specially weak electrolytes give maximum number of ions at infinite dilution, then Homoeopathic drugs cannot be an exception to the rule. Hence these drugs are assumed to be in the ionised state and their activation on the tongue and experiences of med- icinal effect by the nervous system of the patient are claimed.

The above explanation is not free from objection as this is not a generalised explanation. Firstly, all Homoeopathic drugs are not electrolytes. Organic substances are generally molecu- lar in nature, sometimes only a few of them exhibit partial electrolytic character. Secondly, in case of potency 12 and onwards one fails to claim the existence of original drug mole- cule or atom as detailed below. Hence application of idea of ionisation does not appear to be helpful in solving the problem.

(2)   Idea of real (practical) Molecule and Physicist's Molecule :
In order to understand the actual nature of the problem, let us
go into the details of some simple and approximate mathematical calculations to know the number of molecules present in one
drop of the mother tincture and any potentised drug. Before
making the above calculation, for convenience of the reader of
this book, let us calculate number of molecules present in one
drop of water.

(a)   The volume of 2 drops of water is 0.1 c.c. hence the
volume of 1 drop of water is 0.05 c.c.

(b)   The number of molecules present in a mole is called
Avogadro's number (N), the value of this is $6x10^{23}$
approximately which is a constant.

(c)   Weight of one more of water = 18 gms.
Density of water is taken as 1.

$$As\ Density = \frac{Mass}{Volume}$$

$$or\ Volume = \frac{Mass}{Density}$$

Hence volume of 1 mole of water i.e. 18 gms. of water
= 18/1 c.c. = 18 c.c.

(d)   Now, number of molecules contained by 1 mole or
18 c.c. water is = $6x10^{23}$

Therefore, number of molecules contained by 1 drop of
water

i.e. 0.05 c.c. water = $\frac{6x10^{23}}{18}$ x 0.05

$$= \frac{0.05 \times 10^{23}}{3}$$ = 0.016 x 10^{23} (approx)

= 1.6 x 10^{21} (approx.)

Coming to the case of Homoeopathic drugs, let us
calculate the result exactly in a similar way as done above in the
case of water. But here, there are some difficulties. Weight of
one mole of drug and its density will differ from drug to drug.
Hence we have to make some approximations. We take some
extreme cases.

Case (I) Assumed that the weight of one mole of the

original drug is 500 gms. and its density is 0.5.

Hence volume of 1 mole of original drug

$$= \frac{500}{0.5} \text{ c.c.} = 1000 \text{ c.c.}$$

Now, 1000 c.c. of original medicine contains 6×10^{23} molecules. Hence 1 drop or 0.05 c.c. of original medicine contains

$$\frac{6 \times 10^{23} \times 0.05}{1000} \text{ molecules} = .30 \times 10^{20} \text{ molecules}$$
$$= 0.03 \times 10^{21} \text{ molecules}.$$

Case (II) Assumed that the weight of one mole of the original drug is 200 gms. and its density is 1.

Hence volume of 1 mole of original drug

$$= \frac{200 \text{ c.c.}}{1} = 200 \text{ c.c.}$$

Now, 200 c.c. of original medicine contains 6×10^{23} molecules. Hence 1 drop or 0.05 c.c. of original medicine contains

$$\frac{6 \times 10^{23}}{200} \times 0.05 \text{ molecules} = \frac{.30}{2} \times 10^{21} \text{ molecules}$$

$$= 0.15 \times 10^{21} \text{ molecules}$$

So we have seen,

1 drop of water contains 1.6×10^{21} molecules.

1 drop of original drug in the case I contains 0.03×10^{21} molecules. Whereas in the case II contains 0.15×10^{21} molecules.

Hence we can represent this result in a general way that 1 drop of original drug contains $N \times 10^{21}$ molecules where value of $n = 0.01$ to 3 or so.

Hence one drop of a drug of potency 11 contains

$10^{-22} \times n \times 10^{21}$ molecules $= n/10$ molecules.

Hence 1 drop of a Homoeopathic drug having potency II contains hardly an atom of the original drug.

What about the higher potency ? From 12 onward the drugs do not appear to contain original drug atom or molecule on the basis of above calculation, now how they work ?

The above result is obtained when the value of Avogadro's

number (N) is taken as 6×10^{23} approximately. Some people even doubt the above value of Avogadro's number. They are of the opinion that when both lower and higher potencies are curative, then it is not proper to accept the idea that Homoeo drug in higher attenuations are devoid of original drug molecules or atom. Hence they claim that real molecules found out by Homoeopaths are different from the physicist's molecules.

It may be noted that the above value of Avogadro's number is the mean value of a number or determinations following different methods. The most accurate value of Avogadro's number is taken as 6.023×10^{23}. Hence Scientists and Homoeopaths differ in their opinions, though both parties are equally strong on the basis of their experimental findings.

(3) **The idea of the existence of micromolecules of substances in the intermolar spaces** : In order to account for the deviation as already discussed above, an idea of the existence of "Micromolecules" or "dilutes" of substances in the intermolecular spaces has been postulated in recent years. These micromolecules are supposed to be isotopic in character being identical in electronic number and configuration of their atoms but at the same time insignificantly small in relative rest masses being devoid of protons and neutrons.

The net negative charge in the micro-atom is further supposed to be counter balanced by net positive charge in the nucleus consisting of the same number of positrons accompanied possibly with same infinitely small neutral particles. Due to their comparatively insignificant masses, the particles (dilute) may by well assumed to be far beyond the limit of Avogadro's number (N).

At the first glance the above explanation appears to have little weight, but when we think of its validity in the whole range of dilution (from 1 to MM), it fails to satisfy us. The presence of micromolecules only in the limited intermolecular spaces are not expected to be sufficient enough to meet the objections raised above, specially the presence of drug particles in the case of higher and highest potency. Further the above explanation is not a generalised one. One fails to understand the applicability of the above explanation only in the case of Homoeopathic dilutions whereas the dilution of general electrolytes are not affected on the same basis.

(4)   The idea of cybernetics or theory of information :
As already discussed above, to explain the reactivity of Homoeopathic dilution is a controversial subject. Hence a section of thinkers try to solve the problem in a different light. They take the help of Cybernetics which is a branch of Science. 'Cybernetics' is also called theory of information. The information of the presence of particular entity can be given to the concerned agency only with the help of certain energy. When a drop of medicine of potency 11 is mixed with 99 drops of alcohol and 10 strokes are given to the resulting mixture which is a medicine of the 12th potency, the information of a portion of medicine present in potency 11 reaches the medicine or potency 12 in presence of certain energy in the form of 10 strokes.   In a similar way the activity of higher potencies are also explained with the help of 'cybernetics or theory of information'.

The potentised Homoeopathic medicine acts on the patient through his Aura or Bioplasmic body when it is transmitted from a distance.

CHAPTER VI

PRINCIPLE INVOLVED IN TRANSMISSION OF HOMOEO DRUG ENERGY FROM A DISTANCE

OR

THE MECHANISM OF DRUG TRANSMISSION

An attempt is being made to explain the principle involved in transmission of Homoeo drug energy from a distance. The actual mechanism of the process is discussed in Art. 10 of this chapter. A knowledge of relevant ideas expressed in Arts. 1 to 9 is essential in order to follow the Art. 10. So for the convenience of the reader, Arts. 1 to 9 have been written in short, they do not present any detailed account of the topic discussed.

Electromagnetic Wave

(1) The electromagnetic wave theory was firstly proposed by Clark Maxwell in 1864 in order to explain the behavior of light. According to this theory, light is considered as the result of rapidly alternating displacement currents in the medium which give rise to magnetic effects, similar to those associated with conduction currents. The two fields, the electric and the magnetic, inseparably associated, the one varying proportionately with the other and the variation of one giving rise to the other, urge each other forward with a finite velocity viz. that of light. The fact that mutually perpendicular electric and magnetic fields are always confined to a plane perpendicular to the direction of propagation accounts very well for the transverse nature of the light waves replacing the vibration of "mechanical ether" of the older wave theory.

(2) The superiority of the electromagnetic theory over the mechanical theory of light was soon fully recognised because—

    (a) It enabled the velocity of light to be deduced from purely electromagnetic measurements.

(b) By its very nature it allowed only transverse plane light waves.

(3) Maxwell proposed his theory, but electromagnetic waves were not actually produced and detected at that time. His theory received a direct experimental confirmation in 1888 when Hertz produced electromagnetic waves from an oscillatory electric current. Hertz demonstrated that-

(a) Electromagnetic waves are much longer than light waves.

(b) These waves could be reflected, refracted, focussed by a lens, polarised and so on. In short they exhibited properties similar to those of light.

(c) These waves obey all the laws applicable to light waves. Hence these waves (like light waves) on meeting a plane surface normally suffer transmission, reflection or absorption simultaneously.

(d) These waves are propagated in free space with the same velocity as that of light.

(e) There is existence of electromagnetic waves even in vacuum also.

(f) Electromagnetic waves do not require any medium for propagation or transmission (for example, light travels from sun to earth through space which does not contain any material medium. Similarly, radio waves are transmitted through empty space). From these evidences it was concluded that light consisted of electromagenetic waves.

4. (a) All types of electromagnetic radiations travel with the same velocity (V). They differ form one another, however, in their wave lengths and, therefore, in frequencies.

(b) The atoms and molecules contain electrical charges, the vibrations of which send out electromagnetic radiations. The electromagnetic waves emitted by atoms and molecules cover a very wide range of frequencies of wave-lengths forming a long gamut of radiations which is known as electromagnetic spectrum shown in the chart below.

Electromagnetic Spectrum Chart

Electromagnetic radiation.	Wave length		Frequency (Sec.$^{-1}$)
	(in A^0)	(in Cm.)	
Radio waves	3×10^{14} to 3×10^7	3×10^6 to 3×10^{-1}	1×10^{14} to 1×10^{11}
Infrared	3×10^7 to 7600	3×10^{-1} to 7.6×10^{-5}	1×10^{11} to 4×10^{11}
Visible	7600 to 3800	7.6×10^{-5} to 3.8×10^{-5}	4×10^{14} to 7.5×10^{14}
Ultraviolet	3800 to 1	3.8×10^{-5} to 1×10^{-8}	7.6×10^{14} to 3×10^{18}
X-ray	100 to 0.01	1×10^{-6} to 1×10^{-10}	3×10^{16} to 3×10^{20}
Gamma rays	0.1 to 0.0001	1×10^{-9} to 1×10^{-12}	3×10^{19} to 3×10^{22}
Cosmic ray	0.001 to Zero	1×10^{-11} to Zero	3×10^{21} to infinite

The above chart shows that :-

(i)   Electromagnetic radiations cover a very wide range of wave lengths, viz., from less than $0.001 A^0$ to $3 \times 10^{14} A^0$ and hence frequencies from 1×10^{11} to infinite.

(ii)   Thus, human eye can detect electromagnetic radiations in a short range of $3800 A^0$ to $7600 A^0$ only.

5.   Not only atoms or molecules of elements, but even a single electron subjected to a periodic motion would send out a train of electromagnetic waves i.e. radiate energy. If the charge, initially at rest, is given a sudden jerk i.e. a positive acceleration, or if initially in motion it is suddenly stopped i.e. given a negative acceleration a single electromagnetic pulse is sent out, analogous to the sound pulse or crack emitted when a steel ball collides with a massive steel plate. If the acceleration be such that the charge vibrates back and forth along a linear path or moves at uniform speed along a circular path (both are cases of simple harmonic oscillators) a train of electromagnetic waves is given out analogous to the sound waves sent out by a vibrating tuning fork.

6.   As discussed above, electromagnetic radiation is a form of energy. The energy gained depends upon the frequency of the radiation absorbed. Greater is the frequency (i.e. shorter the wavelenth) of the radiation absorbed, greater is the gain in energy. Thus a radiation in ultraviolet region has much greater energy than that in visible region. Similarly, a radiation in visible region has a higher energy than that in the infrared region.

Raman Effect

7. (a) When a substance is irradicated with monochromatic light, Scattered light is observed in a direction at right angles to that of the incident beam. The frequency of the scattered radiations is generally the same as that of the incident radiation as seen spectroscopically. This type of scattering is known as Rayleigh scattering.

(b) Raman discovered in 1928 that if a light of definite frequency is passed through any substance in the gaseous, liquid or solid state, the light scattered at right angles contains lines not only of the original frequency but also of some other frequencies which are generally lower and only occasionally higher than the frequency of the incident light. The lines of lower frequencies are called Stoke's lines while those of higher frequencies are called anti-stoke's lines. The difference between the incident frequency and the scattered frequency is constant. It is called Raman frequency and it is characteristic of the substance exposed to light and is completely independent of the frequency of the incident light. The amount of light scattered in this way is very small and it can be studied by means of a spectrometer with photographic attachment after prolonged exposure ranging from 8 to 100 hours. This alteration in frequency is known as the Raman effect and it is a very general phenomenon.

(c) The details of the Mechanism and application of Raman effect may be seen in any text-book where this topic is discussed. But it will not be out of place to mention that an insight into ionisation of electrolyte can also be obtained from Raman spectrum. As for example, nitric acid (conc. solution in water) has a Raman Line corresponding to frequency 1310 cm^{-1}. No such frequency is present in sodium nitrate but it is present in nitrous acid (conc.solution). Organic nitro compounds have also a frequency of 1400 cm^{-1}. Hence it is likely that both sodium nitrite and conc. nitric acid have a nitro group-NO_2. In sodium nitrite this is present as an iron while in the nitro compound it is present as an undisassociated molecules, on the other hand, when conc. nitric acid is diluted the Raman Line corresponding to 1310cm^{-1}. fades out and a line at about 1046 cm^{-1}. Displacement appears with increasing intensity. This latter line is due to nitrate iron as has also been obtained with various crystals or solutions of nitrate.

Hair And Wool

8.   (a)   **Chemical Structure :**

Animal fibres like hair, wool and silk are made up of proteins. They do not give such sharp diffraction patterns as does cellulose (cotton being purest form of Cellulose), nevertheless, the photographs are definite enough to show a fibre structure and to permit the dimensions of the unit cell to be determined. Observations of exceptional interest were made by W.T. Astbury (1930) on hair and wool. In the natural state these substances, and animal hairs generally, give almost the same X-ray diffraction pattern, attributed to oriented crystallites of the protein keratin. When the animal hairs are stretched, however, the positions of spots are completely changed although the X-ray photograph retains the characteristic of fibre pattern, which now bears a striking resemblance to that for silk. In the unstretched or α-state the unit of structure repeats itself every 5.1A^0., but in the stretched or β-state the repetition occurs after 3.4A^0. Since the X-ray pattern of the latter form of keratin resembles that of fibre, it is probable that β-keratin consists of a chain of amino acid (-NHCHCHR.) residue. In the natural hair or wool fibre the chains are linked by bridges of sulphur atoms i.e. s-s, in cystine, which can be obtained form keratin.

In fibroin each repeating unit consists of two amino acid residues, and so the spacing is approximately twice that in β keratin. The original views concerning the structure of α keratin are now known to be unsatisfactory, and it is probable that this substance occurs in the form of a folded spiral with three amino acid residues to each turn of the spiral;

this would account for the observed spacing of $5.1A^0$. Upon exerting a tension on the α keratin, the spiral presumably uncoils, thus leading to the long-chain β-form. It is of great interest to mention that if the stretching load is removed β keratin returns to the α form, but if the fibre is exposed to steam while being stretched, more or less permanent set is acquired in the extended form. However, moisture and heat, without the application of tension, result in a tendency to return to the coiled structure. These observations have been used to account for such familiar phenomena as "permanent wave" of hair, and the creasing and shrinkage of woolen materials.

(b) **Charges :-** Animal fibres like wool are amphoteric in nature and the charge on the fibre is readily altered by adjustment of PH of the medium. A direct evidence in support of amphoteric nature of wool fibres is that these fibres are dyed by both positive and negative dye stuffs by shifting the PH of the medium.

DILUENTS

9.   It is well known that there are mainly three diluents which are used in the preparation of Homoeopathic remedies :-

(i)   Sugar of milk or lactose (C_{12} H_{22} O_{11} H_2O)

(ii)   Ethyl alcohol (C_2 H_5 OH)

(iii) Water (H_2O)

These substances are said to be inert as they have no medicinal properties at all. D.S. Rawson's view regarding the dilution of remedy may be emphasized at this point. He is considering the magnitude of radiation effect on homoeopathic remedies giving a simple mathematical calculation. Let us consider a system is which Rm. Solute molecules are reacting and let total no. of molecules present in the system be Sm. Hence fraction of solute molecules which react=Rm/Sm. Now, as the solution becomes more and more dilute, Sm is tending to zero, hence Rm/Sm goes on increasing; hence he has concluded that the magnitude of the radiation effect can be said to increase with dilution. This view of his is really concomitant with the principle of homoeopathic philosophy as he has remarked.

10. Principle Involved In Transmission Of Homoeo Drug Energy From A Distance

EXPERIMENTS :-

A number of experiments have been made to study the effect of transmission of homoeo drug energy from a distance and the influence of the drug energy on patients kept at a distance has been proved beyond doubt in all these experiments, establishing the reliability of the method. The experiments may be summed up as follows :-

1. As discussed already, on page 26, we have seen that the percussion note made on the chest of a man changed when another man approached him with an open vial containing sulphur 200, the distance between the two persons being about twelve metres.

2. In another set of experiments, it was thought worth while to test the influence of medicine on patients placed at a distance using only their belongings like hair, blood, signature, photograph, voice etc. and the medicine either in direct contact or placed at a distance within certain limits.

   (a) Transmission By Nerve :-

   In many cases when the medicated globule is placed in the hands of patients, they feel relief as transmission takes place via the nerve of the hand.

   (b) Transmission Through Blood :-

   The haemorrhage of a patient kept at a distance was checked by making contact of the blood stain (obtained on a cloth or paper, of the same escaping blood) with the appropriate remedy.

   (c) Transmission Through Hair :-

   In majority of experiments patient's hair has been used, no matter whether the patient is a man, women, or an animal such as a cow, buffalo, dog, cat etc. So far as the use of medicine is concerned, it is used in conventional forms (i) one medicated globule (ii) small amount of medicated sugar of milk (iii) aqueous solution of medicated powder or liquid.

   MEDICINE :- Using any form of medicine mentioned above the hair is brought in contact with the medicine and the patient kept at a distance experiences its effect. In practice the use of aqueous solution of medicated globule or powder or liquid medicine is very convenient as it can be readily prepared in one dram phial. Then a hair of the patient is inserted into the solution, the phial well corked, keeping a portion of the hair outside the phial, and 10 strokes are given to the phial.

Further, it has also been seen that it is not essential to place hair and medicine in contact together. The hair kept at a certain distance from the medicine produces the same effect as when it is in direct contact. In case of aggravation, the hair is detached and amelioration starts after certain period. But in case of improvement or amelioration transmission is continued.

A number of experiments have been made using hair (see Chapter "Experimental observations" of this book and many others reported by a section of workers which may be seen in Homoeopathic Journals) because this method is convenient.

(d)   Transmission Through Signature Or Photo-graph :-

In some cases signature or writing or photograph of the patient has been used. When a selected remedy is put on the signature or writing or photograph of the patient, it affects him (patient) at once. A number of experiments have been made successfully. Please see pages 67 and 68.

(e)   Transmission Through Sound :-

(i)   Using a telephone and (ii) A tape-recorder.

A patient narrates his trouble on telephone and the doctor opens the cork of the phial of appropriate remedy during conversation with the patient, relief is felt by the patient instantaneously.

To further check the effect of transmission through sound a taperecorder has been used in one case. During the production of sound of the patient by this instrument, the cork of appropriate remedy was opened and the patient at a distance felt relief.

All these experiments force any one to believe that it is not necessary for a patient to take appropriate remedy orally to restore health, the goal can be reached safely by transmission of homoe drug energy from a distance through any natural belonging to the patients.

(ii) Explanation :-

To offer satisfactory explanation of the phenomena observed is the next question. In view of the fact that the effect of transmission on the patient's body is very quickly observed (even in seconds), no matter whatever be distance between the patient and the place of transmission, it may be believed that there is ejection of some sort of characteristic radiation or wave with extremely high velocity from the appropriate medicine and the belonging to the patient such as hair etc. facilitates in some way or other the transmission of that curative radiation up to the patient. Again for the cure of the patients, it is essential that they should be exposed to the above mentioned radiation or wave, continuously for a desired length of time and hence there should be some device to control the time for which the radiation is transmitted.

About the nature of radiation or wave, it will not be out of place to mention that it cannot be a sound wave or thermal radiation. Sound travels with a velocity of 1120 ft. per second only, and after travelling a very short distance the sound-wave appears to be decaying practically. Further, there is no source in the experiment, which is continuously producing sound-wave or thermal wave for the desired length of time. Hence radiation should be essentially electromagnetic. With this idea in mind the following assumptions are made to explain the process of transmission of Homoeo drug energy from a distance.

(a) Assumptions :-

(1) Electromagnetic waves are incident on medicine at infinite number of planes and they are scattered at right angles to the direction of incidence.

(2) The scattered radiations have a different frequency from the incident radiation and the difference in frequency between the above radiations is the characteristic of the medicine used, but it is independent of the incident radiation.

(3) Initially the patient's body and the patients's belonging such as hair, etc. have got the same frequency of vibration but as soon as the patient's belongings are placed in the sphere of influence or field of the medicine, they attain the frequency of the scattered radiation and simultaneously the patients kept at distance also attain almost a similar

frequency (it may be even same frequency) due to forced vibration or sympathetic vibration.

(4)   For the cure of a patient, exposure to radiation with a definite frequency range is needed.

(5)   The time of exposure varies from patient to patient depending on the depth of the disease, rate of improvement, vital force of the patient and other similar factors.

(b)   Validity Of The Assumptions And Explanation of the Method With Criticism :

In the first assumption, mainly two ideas have been expressed :-

(i)   Incidence of electromagnetic waves on medicine at infinite number of planes.

(ii)   Scattering of these waves at right angles to the direction of incidence.

About the first idea one may ask-where from these electromagnetic waves come? The answer is very simple. The reader is referred to Art. 3 of this chapter where various properties of electromagnetic waves are discussed. It is clear that there is existence of electromagnetic waves even in vacuum also (vide Art. 3e). The general laws for reflection, absorption, transmission etc. which are applicable in case of light waves are also applicable in case of electromagnetic waves (vide Art. 3 b). Hence assumption regarding incidence of electromagnetic waves from all directions at infinite number of planes is really not an assumption, rather it is a reality.

Further reason of stressing so much on electromagnetic waves may be questioned. Why do we not consider light waves in place of electromagnetic waves? Even this question does not arise when one knows that light consisted of electromagnetic waves (vide Art. 2). Apart from this, it may be stated that during the experiments on transmission medicinal phials attached with hair were placed either in diffused light or in a drawer in both the cases the patient was influenced. Hence the word 'light' was not dragged in the postulate.

By assuming the incidence of electromagnetic waves, we mean the incidence of radiation in the frequency range 1×10^{11} to infinite as the electromagnetic spectrum chart shows (see page 107). Hence any radiation with desired frequency within above limit may be assumed to be incident on the medicine.

About the second idea expressed above, one may ask the justification of assumption regarding scattering of these waves only at right angles to the direction of incidence. For that the reader is referred to Art. 7 (a) and 7 (b) both. Using light of any frequency the scattering of light by any substance at right angles to the direction of incidence goes by the name of Rayleigh scattering as discussed in Art. 7(a), whereas using light of definite frequency scattering a light at the same angle by a substance is called Raman Effect as discussed in Art. 7(b). In the latter case the scattered radiation has got a different frequency from the incident one and the frequency difference called Raman frequency characteries the substance. In view of the fact that electromagnetic waves behave in the same way as light the assumption regarding scattering of radiation at right angles to the direction of incidence is justified. Hence assumption no.2, is also an established fact.

In the light of these discussions, the path of the incident and scattered radiation can be shown diagrammatically as follows :-

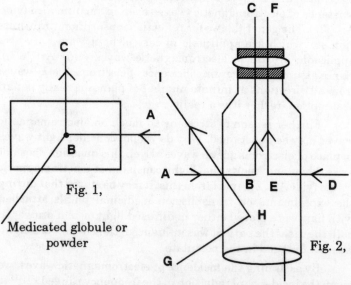

Fig. 1,

Medicated globule or powder

Fig. 2,

Phial containing aqueous solution of medicine

In figure 1, a medicated globule or sugar of milk is placed on a piece of paper. A beam of electromagnetic wave represented by AB is incident on the medicine and scattered at right angles to the direction of incidence which is represented by BC. The path is indicated by the arrow. In a similar way, electromagnetic waves may be assumed to be incident from all possible directions and they are scattered at right angles to the direction of incidence.

In figure 2, a phial containing aqueous solution of the medicine has been shown. Only three beams of electromagnetic waves have been shown in figure. AB represents incident beam whereas EF represents scattered beam, in a similar way GH represents incident beam and HI represents scattered beam and so on. In this way one can understand that there is incidence and scattering of electromagnetic waves in infinite no. of planes.

Even after this detailed discussion, if one hesitates to accept the scattering of the electromagnetic waves essentially at right angles to the direction of incidence, it may be said that by assuming the scattering at any angle to the direction of inci-dence the final result remains the same i.e. there is incidence and scattering of electromagnetic waves in infinite no. of planes.

Further, the reader is referred to Art.5 according to which atoms, molecules, even single electron on jerking radiate elec-tromagnetic waves. The phial containing medicine is given jerk during transmission, hence ejection of electromagnetic waves are always expected.

Now coming to the third assumption one may note the result of modern forensic science study, according to which though two faces may be similar in appearance the striations of fingers and hairs of one individual differ from those of the other individual and these striations and hairs may have a specific relation with the body of that particular individual. The hair of a particular man represents the same constitution in a mini-ature form, of which the particular man is himself made of. The hair has got the same characteristic vibration as that of the body of the individual and this capacity of vibration, capacity to receive and transmit energy of a particular quality is un-changed, even after the hair or any natural belonging to the patient used in these experiments is separated from the body. So initially the patient's body and patient's belonging such as hair etc. have got the same frequency of vibration. When hair or patient's belonging is placed in the field of medicine, the former attains the same frequency as the scattered radiation, which is characteristic of medicine used. Now, attainment of the same frequency by a table as the frequency of a vibrating tuning fork is well known when the stem of the vibrating fork is placed on the top of a table and it is an example of forced vibration.

In a similar way, as soon as the patient's belonging such as hair attains the frequency of vibration of the scattered radiation, simultaneously the patient kept at a distance also attains almost similar (it may be even the same) frequency of vibration due to forced vibration or sympathetic vibration. The effect is instantaneous because radiating involved is electromagnetic one which has got the same velocity as that of light i.e. 186000 miles per second (vide Art. 3 d), hence distance is no bar so far as the immediate observation of the effect of transmission is concerned.

The practical aspect of the 4th and 5th assumptions is so clear to our Homeoeopath brethren that they need not be discussed in detail. One Knows it well that a patient may be cured using appropriate remedy in the potency 6 or 30 or 200 or any other. Whereas other patient may not be cured unless 50 M or C.M potency is used. Hence one can very well agree that for a cure of a patient exposure to radiation within a definite frequency range is needed which is maintained by placing the patient's belonging in the remedy within a definite potency range. Hence no objection can be raised against the 4th assumption.

About the 5th assumption also, no disagreement should be voiced by any one because he knows that in the old process single dose of remedy cures one patient, but a no. of doses of the same remedy may be required for the other patient depending on the condition of the patient.

(c) Indications :-

The effect of transmission on the patient kept at a distance is indicated in various ways as given below :-

(1) Change of temperature of hand and other parts of the body just after transmission is frequently observed in 95% cases.

(2) Aggravation or amelioration in pain if there be any.

(3) Pulse rate or rate of heart beating may change.

(4)   Sweat on the face or any part of the body may appear or vanish.

(5)   One may feel thirst or mouth may start watering if dry.

(6)   One may begin to sneeze, cough or yawn or may be sleepy.

(7)   A tingling sensation, sensation of coldness or heat on forehead or any where.

(8)   One may feel giddiness, heaviness, lightness or chill.

(9)   A change in sensation in any part of the body.

(10) Smell of spirit or sensation of spirit in throat.

(11) Change in blood pressure.

(12) Change in taste of mouth.

(13) One may lose sense for sometimes or have fits.

(14) Some may feel nervousness or be hilarious.

(15) One may feel urge for urine or stool or their urges may vanish

(16) Tendency to scratch or stretch body, rub limbs or crack joints.

(17) Feeling of formications

(18) Feeling of intoxiation etc.

(d)   **The above Mechanism of Transmission also Explains the Following Facts :-**

(1)   It is not essential that the hair or any other belonging to the patient placed in direct contact with medicine. Even if it be placed a certain distance apart, the action will be similar to that when it is in direct contact. Because the main thing is to place the patient's belonging well within the field of medicine, so that the scattered radiation may be received by the patient's belonging.

(2)   In the oral method of administration of drug, the same mechanism as discussed above is operative. When globule is placed on the tongue of the patient, the scattered radiation is directly received by the patient's body through the nerve of tongue.

(3)   When the medicine is placed in the hands or between tips of fingers or any other parts of the body the patient is in direct contact of the medicine (not essentially the tongue) and in all those cases the scattered radiation is directly

received by the nerve of that limb.

(4) Transmission of the drug energy through sound of the patient on telephone or tape recorder is also explained following the same mechanism. Here the sound received the scattered radiation, and patient at a distance is affected.

(5) Lastly it may be noted that the above discussed process of transmission is a continuous process which is also explained by the proposed mechanism. Experimental evidence in support of this fact is also known. A person was exposed to the radiation for one year during the course of his treatment for certain trouble. He was free form the trouble but he did not report. After one year he reported heaviness of his head, pain in the whole body etc. Then his hair was detached from the medicine and at the same time telephonic contact was also made. The patient felt relief at once and within a few days he was perfectly alright. It may be noted that the distance between the patient and the place of transmission was about two hundred kilometers. Though it has not been seen experimentally, however it is expected that a patient broadcasting at a radio station may be affected simultaneously with the opening of medicine phial near a radio or transistor set.

CHAPTER VII

TECHNIQUE AND METHOD OF DRUG TRANSMISSION

The potentised Homoeopathic drug is a kind of energy and alcohol, globule or sugar of milk is only a vehicle which stores and carries that energy as already mentioned in the previous chapter. A drug cannot be called Homoeopathic unless it is selected according to principles and matched in its vibratory plane with that of the sick person. Being in the form of energy the drug can be administered to the patient in various ways not essentially, orally. Broadly the method of administration of drug can be divided into two parts - (1) Direct method and (2) Indirect method. The method in which the drug is brought in direct contact with the patient or any link is established between the drug and the patient, is called direct method, as for example : (a) Oral (b) Tactual (c) Olfactory and (d) Telephonic. Let us explain each of the direct method in details.

(a)   Oral :

Oral method may be called traditional method as it has been used since the very inception of Homoeopathy. The patient is administered on his tongue a few medicated tiny sugar globules, or is given a drop of the drug in a little quantity of sugar of milk or in a dram phial containing distilled water for a dose. But the author would usually administer a single tiny medicated pill or globule for a dose prior to this discovery of his. It is generally assumed that drug should be swallowed down but it is not essential. The very contact of drug with the nerves of the tongue is sufficient to activate the economy of the patient. This is simply putting a drug in the electromagnetic field of the patient.

(b)   Tactual :

In this method, the drug is brought in close contact with the patient or rubbed in on his or her skin. Samuel

Hahnemann says in his "chronic diseases part I", "If this same remedy that has been found useful is at the same time in its watery solution rubbed in (even in small quantities) one or more parts of the body which are most free from the morbid ailments (i.e. on an arm or on the thigh or leg which has neither cutaneous eruptions, nor pains or cramps) then the curative effects are much increased". Here also it may be noted that the drug energy is put in the field of the patient. The author sometimes asks the patient to hold one tiny medicated globule between tips of fingers and observe the effect. The effect is felt at once. Generally it is done to test the correctness of the remedy or potency whenever there is shortage of time or absence of hair though this practice is harmful and so discouraged.

(c)   Olfactory :

Long long ago the author sometimes used to hold an open medicinal vial near the nose of the unconscious patient and he or she opened eyes immediately. In this connection he has the support of the father of Homoeopathy who has written in his "Chronic disease" smelling of an opened vial where in one or more such pettels are contained, proves itself the smallest and weakest dose with the shortest period of duration in its effects". Here too the aura of the patient is influenced by the drug energy.

The above three methods are traditional methods.

(d)   Telephonic :

There is yet another direct method called by the author "Telephonic". He has experimented successfully and it is quite distinct from the traditional methods. In this method the drug and the patient at a distance are linked together through the medium of sound via telephone wire. That is why it is called a direct method. In this method the vial containing the required drug is opened and held up close to the receiver while taking talking to the patient on phone. The vibration of the voice of the patient comes in contact with the vibration of the drug energy and thereby brings the patient under the influence of the drug. Here too, the electromagnetic field of the patient is influenced by the drug energy.

Indirect Method

The methods in which there is no direct link between the patient and the drug are called indirect. It may be called wireless in the medical field. The patient acts as a receiving set and the doctor acts as an operator. This human set is very sensitive and has got two way traffic it receives as well as sends off radiations.

Like direct method, this is also applied in different ways, as for examples :

(a)   Through any natural belonging to the patient i.e. detached hair, blood stains, sputum etc.

(b)   Through the photograph of the patient.

(c)   Through the signature or hand-writing of the patient.

(d)   Recorded voice of the patient on tape etc. when any thing belonging to the patient say his photograph, signature or his voice is brought in contact with the drug, the patient is thus brought immediately under the influence of the drug. The distance between the patient and the drug is no barrier whatsoever.

Transmitting Set

The vial or the container of drug along with drug and any of the above media of transmission is called "Transmitting set".

The process of transmission of drug as a whole is called "Sahni Transmission" and its effect on the patient is termed as the "Sahni Effect".

Keeping in view the convenience of the patient and the doctor, the hair is probably the best among all the indirect media used for drug transmission. The hair can easily be kept in constant physical touch with the drug solution prepared in one dram phial. The method of application is very simple and handy. The patient's hair is put on a book or in folds of a register and one tiny globule of a selected drug is simply brought in contact with one end of the detached hair of the patient. The drug in liquid or powder form is also used. In the beginning of discovery this method was used but gradually another method was evolved for convenience. In this method one medicated globule is dissolved in distilled water and one end of the detached hair is inserted into the phial containing above solution and it is well corked so that the other end of that hair may float in the air serving as an antenna. It is not essential that one end of the hair should remain out side the phial. Even if the hair is submerged into the phial, it works without any hindrance because the radiation is of electromagnetic nature, but keeping one end of the hair outside the phial is in general practice due to convenience in handling it. The phial is in general practice due to convenience in handling it. This phial containing the drug and hair (Transmitting set) is given 10 strokes (succussions) to enhance the action of the drug. This transmitting set is not handed over to the patient concerned as it was done previously, which is mentioned in the first edition of the book. It is kept in the author's chamber and the patients send reports through letters, telegrams, telephone etc. in case of aggravation but in normal course they come to the author every month on fixed dates or send monthly reports when they do not turn up. In case of aggravation it is not essential to detach hair at once. It should be watched. In majority of cases Homoeopathic aggravation subsides without detaching. This set has an advantage over the use of dry globule or powder as it is easy to maintain contact of the hair with the drug in aqueous solution for a longer period and also the plussing is easily done.

The hair can be obtained by uprooting from the head or any part of the body, or chopping off a portion of it with a pair of scissors. The hair can be inserted into the phial by either ends (of the hair). A hair once taken may be used repeatedly for the same or different drugs or potencies, so long as it has its physical existence intact.

Transmitting Set "On" or "Off"

When the hair is inserted into the medicinal solution or brought in contact with the drug, this process is called "On" i.e. the transmitting set was set on. If the hair is detached or taken off the solution of the drug, it is called "Off" i.e. the transmitting set was set off.

Plussing :

In course of treatment sometimes it happens that the good effect of the drug ceases to appear at a certain stage or aggravation sets in, in such conditions some strokes given to the transmitting set brings about the desired effect and in case of no response even after this the potency has to be raised a bit by plussing. To slightly raise the potency, the solution of the T.S. (Transmitting Set) is thrown away and it is refilled with fresh distilled water and 5 or 10 strokes are given to the T.S. This whole process of throwing and refilling is called "Plussing". If this is done once it is called one plus or one plussing. If repeated called two plussings and so on. The hair is then put back into the phial. Generally one plus suffices for the purpose, but even 4, 5 or more plussings may be needed.

Generally the practitioners repeat a certain potency thrice then they switch over to the higher one. The gap between any two potencies is too wide in the following list of potencies 30C, 200C, 1M, 10M, 50M, C.M. etc. so switching over higher potency means too high a jump and this jump may miss the plane where in the disease is harboured (anchored) but in plussing method the chance of missing plane is minimised. With every plussing it has been experienced that the drug reveals its further good effect. Moreover it eliminates the chance of violent reaction. If a single potency is tuned with the vibration of the patient, occasional plussings give a very satisfactory result. If further plussings do not bring about desired effects then only the next higher potency is resorted to. The author rarely repeats the same potency.

Series of Potencies

Regarding the cure of a chronic disease, Dr. J.T. Kent has said, "When we recognise the fact of the long years of existence of chronic cases, also they are often inherited from several generations, if a cure is made in the course of two or three years it is indeed a speedy cure. It takes from two to five years to cure chronic diseases".

The world is advancing rather rapidly and the modern medical therapy has to keep pace with it. People have no patience to undergo long period of treatment for permanent cures. It is rather amusing that they prefer patch-work to long continued permanent cure.

Really time factor is a great problem though the patient as a whole is treated by Homoeopathy. To cut short the duration of treatment to effect a cure one project "Experiment on a series of potencies" at a time was taken by the Research Institute or Sahni Drug Transmission and Homoeopathy under the author's Directorship and the result was found to be encouraging.

There are certain laws and procedures to select a correct remedy for a particular patient but there is none for the selection of right potency that is why there are various opinions and experiences regarding it. Some are high potenists like Dr. Kent while others like Dr. Boericke are low potenists.

It is a matter of long experience to arrive at standard potencies. Administering higher and higher potencies one at a time takes a long period to effect a cure. Generally the depth of a disease is unknown to the physician and a particular potency may miss that plane of the disease. It is just like throwing a net to catch fish under deep water. Hence under this project a series of three potencies as for examples — 30, 200, and 1M; 200, 1M; 1M, 10M and 50M; 10M, 50M and C.M. in different phials are transmitted one after another at a time. If the first potency of the series acts favorably then the rest of the series are not transmitted immediately. Action is watched for a week, fortnight or even a month. Even after a month if every thing goes on well, simply plussing is done so long as it goes on acting. Sometimes a single potency after plussing affects the cure. If next higher potency is needed, it is transmitted through another hair separately, letting the previous one work and the third time still higher is used. Generally one set of lower potency is dropped and the next higher is transmitted. In this way two or three potencies are transmitted in different phials through different hairs at a time. Any serious aggravation has to be guarded against. In case of aggravation the highest is set off first and then the next lower in the series and so on. If aggravation is checked by detaching hair from the highest potency then the rest of the series are not disturbed otherwise all are set off.

While transmitting the first potency of the series, if the action is not detected clearly, in that case the next higher is transmitted and so on. Plussings are generally done in the transmitting sets of a series at intervals according to requirements. Generally patients are called in after a month to report the progress and needful is done. Good results have been obtained in this project and the period of cure is cut short by 25% at present. The project is a new one and more is expected from it in future... In one case of uterine and rectum Cancer a series of potencies has done miracle. Prior to this the patient used to experience bleeding from rectum almost every month for more than a year. After transmitting Puls. 200, 1M and 10M in series bleeding was checked and rapid cure was affected.

CHAPTER VIII

EXPERIMENTAL OBSERVATIONS

Case No. 1

The problem as to how to transmit the Homoeopathic Dynamic Drug-Energy to the ailing human beings had been taxing the author's mind since long. He had no sleep during the night of 5.1.1967 due to the vexing problem in his mind. In the morning of 6.1.1967 Mr. A. Kumar of Bhagalpur came to him for the 2nd time to show his son, Master Pramod Kumar, a student of standard VIII of St. Xavier's H.E. School, Sahebganj, Santal Pragana, who had been suffering from eczema and examined by him on 26.12.1966. After repertorising the case by Kent's Repertory Ars. Alb. was selected and it was administered in the 200th Potency. Mr. A. Kumar himself, a patient of chronic peptic ulcer had been under the Ayurvedic treatment of Dr. R.C. Shastri, who was absent that day. He requested him to give some medicine to get relief of his acute colic pain. A flash came to his mind to try Ars. Alb. 200 on his uprooted hair. Ars. Alb. was selected at random, as sometimes the same remedy helps the blood relations. The author requested him to give a hair from his head and it was done. It was placed on the cover of a book and one globule of Ars. Alb. 200 was brought in contact with the root of his hair. Mr. Kumar uttered, "I am feeling a churning sensation in my abdomen" The author's joy knew no bound. He detached the hair from the medicated globule and pain was reduced to 75% at once. The author was very conscious of psychology at that time. He said, "Well the remaining 25% pain will vanish this time". Instead of using Ars. Alb. 1M he came down to 30 and one drop of it was poured on the root of the same hair. To utter surprise, the pain became intense and he left the author's chamber in agony.

The cup of his joy was full to the brim as the long-standing taxing problem was solved. Since then he began to experiment in each and every case with success.

The author wrote down an article under the caption, "Homoeo. Dynamic Medicines can be transmitted", which was published in the "Torch of Homoeopathy, April 1967 issue, New Colony, Jaipur, Rajasthan with encouraging comments and suggestions by the editor, Dr. Chandra Prakash.

On 30.3.1967 Mr. A. Kumar when he came to the author for his son, narrated that after going from him on 6.1.67 he had become almost unconscious due to intense colic and an allopathic physician was called in for his rescue. He had been confined to bed for a couple of days. But that was the last and most violent attack. He was relieved of his colic after three days and since then he had been free from his obstinate colic.

The 6th Jan. 1967 and Mr. A. Kumar will remain commemorable in the history of DISCOVERY OF TRANSMISSION OF DRUG-ENERGY THROUGH SEPARATED HAIR OF PATIENT.

Case No. 2
Abortion

W/o. Shri R. Singh of Muzaffarpur aged 23, was brought to the author on 6.12.1968 for her treatment as she had been a victim of habitual abortions in third month of pregnancy. She was carrying pregnancy for two months only and was very much apprehensive because the previous two abortions could not be checked in spite of wonderful drugs. Her husband's blood test both Wasserman and V.D.R.L. showed "Positive". The symptoms were very poor still it was repertorized as follows :

(1)   Abortion in third month - Apis, Cimicif. Croc., Eup-P., M.S., Sabina, Sec., Thuja, and ustil.

(2)   Worse Carriage - Croc. and Thuja.

(3)   Aversion to open air - Thuja.

Thuja 1M was transmitted on 6.12.68 and her palms became sweaty. It was kept on till 25.4.69 and detached on 26.4.69 due to cough and cold. From that day some Biochemic medicines were given from time to time till delivery.

She gave birth to a healthy female child at 1.10 A.M. on 4.7.69 in the Bettiah hospital.

Case No. 3
Alopecia

Miss S. Kumari D/o. Sri D.M. Prasad, a govt. employee of Patna, aged 6½, was brought to the author on 14.2.70 for falling of hair for the last ten months. She had been under the treatment of Homoeopaths without any benefit. Hair completely fell from temples, vertex, occiput and eye-brows. There were very small patches of hair left near ears. Her head looked shiny as if completely shaved. The case was repertorised with the following rubrics :

(1)   Habit of putting finger into mouth - C.C., Cham. and Ipecac.

(2)   Likes Sweets - C.C. and Ipecac.

(3)   Dislikes milk - C.C.

C.C. 0/20 was transmitted. Hairs began to grow in a week. On 17.2.70 hair from the medicine was detached by mistake. S.L. was continued till 15.3.70 and on 16.3.70 C.C. 0/20 was again transmitted, which was detached due to cold on 20.3.70. On 7.5.70 it was seen that 80% of hairs had grown. She developed aversion to sweets and left the habit of putting finger into her mouth. Phos 0/20 was transmitted on 7.5.70. Her head and eye-brows are almost full of hair.

Case No. 4
Asthma

S/o. Mr. R.N. Sinha aged 15 months of Patna was brought to the author for treatment of his asthmatic troubles in May, 1967. The following symptoms were noted :

(1)   He was hoarse and had dry hacking cough. Cough was aggravated during sleep.

(2)   Mind-He was peevish and irritable. He was angry and began to strike if anybody touched him.

(3)   Combing was not allowed and had dandruff and itching in scalp.

(4)   Mouth-Tongue clean and red with pimples on sides of it.

(5)   Likes-Salty things and earth.

(6)   Dislikes-Sweets.

(7)   Modalities-Better while riding in a carriage and worse

cold, evening and night, (The case was repertorised by Kent) and N.A. was selected.

(1)   Likes earth-Alum., Calc., Cic., Ferr., N.M., N.A. and N.V.

(2)   Irritable-Alum., Calc., Cic., Ferr., N.M., N.A. and N.V.

(3)   Likes salty things--C.C., N.M. & N.A.

(4)   Better riding N.A.

N.A. 200 one globule no. 10 was transmitted.   Before transmitting he had 97^0F. temperature but after it the temperature rose to 99^0F. It was disconnected and the temperature fell down to 98^0F. Again the hair was connected with that globule and temperature touched 99^0F. and his face became flushed. His father was given some globules of N.A. 200 in a dram phial and directed to connect and disconnect according to his condition.

After a month it was reported that the child was much better and he did not have temperature since then. Cough and cold also vanished. He did not need further transmission.

Case No. 5
Asthma

Dr. D.N. Sah aged 40 of Narhan, Samastipur had been a victim of Asthma since the age of 15. He came to the author on 9.8.72 for treatment. He had the following ailments :

(1)   Breathing trouble with Coryza since 25 years.

(2)   Pain in back since 1 year.

(3)   Eczema in hands, palms, neck, fingers, since 5 years.

(4)   Heels pain since 1 year.

(5)   Vertigo since 2 years.

(6)   Knees pain since 20 years.

(7)   Lumbago since 20 years.

(8)   Filarial lump in right arm since long.

(9)   Wart on head since a year.

Previous ailments and their treatment :

(1)   Tingling in limbs in childhood-treated by an allopath.

(2)   Mumps in childhood-treated by an allopath.

(3)   Injury to his head at 6 years age-profuse bleeding and

senseless for some hours.

(4)   Filaria in young age treated by an allopath.

(5)   Scabies suppressed by external use of ointment.

Father died of Rheumatism and bleeding piles.

Mother alive suffering from asthma since 4 years.

He was married at the age of 18 and his wife suffered from T.B. Glands.

He has 4 daughters, all but the youngest one suffered from T.B. Glands in the Cervical regions.

Mind-Abusive, habit of cursing and swearing, miserly,

Craving for salty things.

Breathing trouble aggravated during sleep while lying and better by fan, bending on back and knee-elbow-position.

Back pain better by pressure.

Joints pain worse on beginning of motion and better by motion.

Bleeding after scratching in eczema.

The treatment was started by transmitting Medor 1M on 9.8.72 and he felt heat in his body and pain in chest just after transmission which disappeared after 5 minutes.

13.9.72 -   1.   No breathing trouble.

2.   Pain in heels.

3.   Back pain better

Transmission was put off the previous set. Medo. 10 M was transmitted and heels pain vanished at once.

13.10.72-   (1)   Filarial attack with severe pain in the right arm for 2 days only from 15.9.77.

(2)   Back pain much better.

(3)   Itching violent.

Transmission of medo. 10M was put off.

With the transmission of psor. IM, its plussings carb. veg. 0/3,200 & its plussing, Ars alb. 0/6 and Tuber. IM from time to time according to symptoms he was cured of all troubles mentioned above except slight eczema by the end of Oct. 1973. The patient became irregular in course of treatment and ultimately he discontinued reporting. His Asthma has not relapsed till today (July 1977). He is leading a healthy life.

Case No. 6
Azospermia

Sri S. Yadava aged 35 of Vaishali was married in 1961 but he was not blessed with any issue. His seminal-fluid was tested on 22-12-71 and 14-4-72 and all sperms 25000 and 50000 per c.c. respectively were found almost dead. He came to the author on 5-1-74 for treatment and he was advised to get a recent report. Family as well as his past history furnished no clue for diagnosis. He had been operated upon his left side Hydrocele in 1962 and had mumps in childhood. The following points were noted :-

Mind :-   Talkative, vindictive, obstinate, abusive and weeping on seeing kith & kin.

Craving for sweets but aversion to sour things. he used to sleep covering his mouth during sleep in all seasons with frightful dreams. He used high pillow.

Lyco. 0/3 was transmitted on 5-1-74 and on 3-2-74 he had cold and cough for two days.

2.   Itching body since 10-1-74

Transmission was continued after one plus.

3-3-74—   he could not get seminal fluid tested. Hence. Lyc. was continued after another plus and advised for test.

7-4-74—   Examination report showed sperm as nil (Azospermia) Detaching from Lyc. 0/3, Sul. 0/12 was transmitted on 12-5-74. Plussing was made and continued till 4-7-74 Seminal test on 5-7-74 also found no sperm.

5-7-74—   Ferr. Met. 0/5 was transmitted and continued after plussing in August and September and Seminal fluid test on 21-10-74 reported "Occasional dead sperms were found".

Again after plussing in the previous transmitting set, it was continued and seminal test on 1-1-75 reported. "Number of sperms 75000. 10% motile after 1/2 hour and 4% after 4 hours".

He passed out two round worms 10 inches long, on 17-6-75. Again after plussing treatment was continued till 28-9-75 but he could not produce seminal test report. he did not turn up after Sept. 75 and the reason could not be known inspite of efforts.

Case No.7

Azospermia

Mr. R. Singh aged 27 of Muzaffarpur District was married in 1967. He was not blessed with any issues in 4 years of married life. Hence his parents were anxious. His wife was put under treatment for the purpose. In course of treatment Mr. Singh's Seminal fluid was examined and no sperm was detected. Hence he was also put under modern treatment for some months and again his semen was examined on 2-9-71 and still no trace of sperm was found.

Mr. Singh came to the author on 5-9-71 for treatment and the following data were collected :-

(1) The Seminal fluid test report—fluid 2 c.c.,

Thin, reaction-alkaline. Not a single sperm either alive or dead was found.

(2) Pain in penis after coition since a year.

(3) Dry Ring-worm on his knee and between thighs for the last 3 years. It was aggravated in the rainy season.

(4) He had breathing trouble for the last three years.

(5) Fidgety.

PREVIOUS AILMENTS WITH TREATMENT

(1) Weak constitution since infancy.

(2) Severe Malaria at the age of 11 and heavy doses of quinine were taken.

(3) Scabies in childhood treated externally.

(4) Injury to scrotum by cycle accident 11 years back.

(5) Injury to spine by beating by his father in rage at the age of 16 years. Since then he had pain in chest and back for some years.

(6) He had frequent attacks of cold and cough and was treated by the modern physician.

(7) He had been a victim of Syphilis some years back and was treated allopathically.

(8) His grand-father died of diabetes and his mother has Leucoderma and nothing worth mentioning was detected in his family.

The case was repertorised in the following way (vide

Kent's repertory and Kishore's Cards).

(1)   Aversion to sour things (acids)—

       Abies can., Bell., Clem., Cocc., Ind., Dros., Fer., Met.,
       Ferr., Mur., Ign., Ind., N.P., N.V., A-Phos., Sabad, Sanic,
       Sulph., Syph. and Tubercul.

(2)   Intolerance of contradictions-Cocc., Ferr. Met., Ign., and
       N.V.

(3)   Abuses of quinine-F. Met. and N.V.

(4)   Fidgety-F.Met.

Ferr. was selected as a similimum and it was transmitted
in the 200th potency on 5-9-71. Sufficient S.L. was given. As
soon as it was transmitted he left a tingling sensation in his
whole head.

25-9-1971—Report—(1) Very painful ulcer in his penis just after
                a few days.

          (2) Itching aggravated.

          (3) Respiratory trouble started from 6-9-71.

          (4) Cold and cough on 15-9-91.

Transmission was put off for some days. Started transmitting again on 11-10-71 after plussing, when he got some relief.
Again eruption on penis aggravated and transmission was put
off. There was some relief in his trouble hence F.Met. IM was
transmitted on 7-11-71 and the transmitting set was handed
over to him with an instruction to detach hair in case of violent
reactions. He faced a violent aggravation and did not turn up
again for treatment. His seminal fluid was tested and sufficient
motile and healthy sperms were found. His wife conceived and
gave birth to a female child on 26-10-72 but unfortunately the
baby died. Again she conceived and gave birth to a healthy
female child, who is okay.

Case No.8

Azospermia

(Male Sterility)

Shri B. Chaudhury, aged 35 years, came to the author for
treatment on 2-4-79. He was married in the year 1947 but had
no issue. He married a second wife in the year 1968 with the
same result. Several reports of examination of his semen showed

absence of sperm.

Report dated 12-5-71 :-

Mode of collection	Masturbation.
Quantity	3 c.c.
Colour	White
Odour	Fragrant.
Reaction	Alkaline
Period between collection and examination	1 hour

Microscopic :-

(1)   Sperm   nil
(Azospersmia)

(2)   Epithelial cells and Pus cells :-   Some

(3)   Epithelial cells   05 : 1

2.   Apart from this he had bleeding piles since five years and had undergone operation 2 years back with no appreciable improvement. Haemorrhage with passing of flatus.

3.   Warts on head and feet.

PERSONAL PREVIOUS HISTORY

1.   Scabies suppressed with external application in childhood

2.   Liver affection in childhood.

3.   Surgical operation of the testicles, 13 years back.

4.   Malaria at young age-Abuse of quinine.

5.   Addicted to wine.

6.   Victim of masturbation at early age.

7.   Measles in childhood.

8.   Vaccinated several times.

Parents :-

Father died of small pox. Mother died in early age.

1.   Brother died after insanity, he had 3 children.

2.   Two brothers died in childhood.

Mental Symptoms :- Quiet disposition and mild. Sympathetic. Good memory.

Head — Wart. Vesicles and dandruff.

Throat — Hoarseness. Weak voice.

Stomach — Desires salty things. Aversion to sweets.

Rectum — Stool soft in morning and hard in the evening. Sits long for stool. Sometimes discharge of pus. Discharge of blood on passing flatus.

Penis — Curved. Strong desire for intercourse.

Sleep — Normal. Takes high pillow. Absence of dream.

Extremities-Restless on sitting. Pain in elbow in cold season.

Bath — Desires bath.

Aggravation — Cold, passing flatus.

The case was repertorised thus with 'Kent' :-

(1)   Kind temperament :- Carl., Caust., Cic., Croc., Ign., Iod., Lyc., Manc.. Nat. c., Nat. M., Nit. Ac, Nuph., Nux. V., Phos., and Puls.

(2)   Aversion to Sweets :- Caust, Nit. Ac., and Phos.

(3)   Sexual passion increased :- Caust, Nit. Ac., and Phos.

(4)   Discharge of blood with flatus :- Phos.

Thus Phorphorus was chosen to be the medicine. Phosphorus had also a place in the male sterility in 'Raue Pathology., Hence Phosphrus 05 was transmitted to him through his hair. Plain globules were given to take every morning and evening.

Report dated 16-4-72— (1) Eruption-vesicles on lips on 6/ 4 and (2) had also cold and cough (3)   Discharge of blood with passing of flatus abated from 8-4-72.

Transmission of Phosphorus 0/5 was allowed to continue. 14-5-72-Report of semen by Ashok Pathological Clinic. Khalifabagh, Bhagalpur, was as follows :-

Quantity- 1 c.c.

Colour- Op. white.

Odour- Normal.

Total number of thin sperms- 1,00,000.

Motility-30mts. after discharge-active- 5%

Sluggish-10%

Dead-85%

After 2 hours-0%, 5%, 95%.

Most of the sperms ill-developed. Extreme Oligo and Asthenospermia. Transmission set was given some strokes and it was transmitted again after one plussing. Plain pills were given to take as before.

16-7-72   (1) Black spot in sputum (2) Discharge of thin pus from rectum (3) Acne on face.

Report of Semen dated 11-7-72 from the same clinic :-

Mode of collection	Masturbation
Quantity	2 c.c.
Colour	Opulent white, thin
Odour	Normal.
Total number	700,000.

	Active	Sluggish	Dead
Motility-After 30 mts.	40%	10%	50%
Motility-After 2 hours	30%	10%	60%

Mostly ill-developed and Weak sperm.

Phosphorus 0/12 was transmitted and plain pills to take.

Report dated 1-8-72 from the same clinic :-

Mode, Quantity, colour and odour as above.

Total number-1,00,000

Motility—After 30 mts.	75%	5%	20%
Ater 2 hours	65%	10%	25%

Most of the sperms healthy.

Acute Oligospermia.

Transmission was allowed to continue as before.

Transmission vial was handed over to the patient with directions.

23-9-72-Transmission was changed over to Phos. 0/15.

30-9-72- (1) Cold and cough, (2) Desire for sweets,

(3) Discharge of pus from rectum.

Transmission was changed over to Arsenic Alb. 0/15.

Report dated 9-10-72 from the same clinic :-

Total number-340,000

Motility—After 35 mts.	40%	10%	50%
After 2 hours	30%	10%	60%

Most of the sperm healthy.

Oligo and Asthenospermia.

Arsenic Alb. 0/15 was retransmitted after one plussing,

19-11-72   (1) Semen was not examined.

    (2) No remission in cough.

    (3) Warts on head peeled off.

    (4) Discharge of pus form rectum.

Transmission was stopped. Only Phytum was given.

1-4-73-   (1) Semen not examined.

    (2) Discharge of pus continued.

    (3) Pain in body and fever from 28-3-73.

    (4) Loss of appetite.

    (5) Desire for sweet.

    (6) Sensitive to heat.

Sulphur 0/3 was transmitted. Feeling of well being.

Phytum was given to take.

After the appearance of sperms in semen both his wives were treated by the author for a few months. The first wife was suffering from tubercular glands and the other had menstrual troubles.

Mr. Chaudhury did not return for treatment after 1-4-73. Treatment of his wives also stopped.

It is not known whether he was blessed with a child.

The main purpose of including this case in this book is to show that the treatment proved capable of producing sperms.

Case No. 9
Bed Wetting

Master Vinod Kumar S/o Dr. L.P.Singh aged 7 was brought to the author on 6-2-70, who had been suffering from bed-wetting since long. The case was repertorised with the help of the following :-

    (1)   Puts fingers into his mouth-Cham., C.C. and Ipecac.

    (2)   Grinding of teeh-C.C. and Cham.

    (3)   Likes salty things-C.C.

C.C. 0/20 was transmitted on 6-2-70. He stopped bed-wettiing on 9-2-70. Hence he was instructed to put the transmission off which was done on 11-2-70. Again the trouble started on 11-3-70. After watching, transmission of C.C. 0/20 was repeated on 22-3-70 and detached on 25-3-70 due to cough and cold. He stopped bed-wetting completely.

Case No. 10
Cancer of Back

Md. Y. (aged 40 years) came to the author on 22-8-67 for treatment of an orange sized tumor on his back, which was continuing for the last one year. At first there was no pain in it, but it turned to be painful for the last one month. The tumor was divided into three lobes and on touch it appeared just like a cauliflower. A local M.B.B.S. physician had administered some homoeo medicines but in vain. He forbade him to go for surgery or a biopsy test. He advised him to consult some experienced Homoeopathic physician. The character of the tumor clearly indicated that it was cancerous.

The following symptoms were taken down :-

(1) Pain in tumor ameliorated by hot application.

(2) Anxiety.

(3) Fear of thunder-storm.

(4) Sympathy.

(5) Aversion to meat and fish.

(6) Desire for cold food.

(7) Cold patient.

He had suffered from skin eruptions in childhood. His father had died in 1953 of asthma, which had shocked him much.

The remedy was selected on the following rubrics :-

    (1) Fear of thunder-storm-Bry., Bor., Her., Lach., N.C., Nat. M., N.A., Phos, Rhod., Sep., Sulph.

    (2) Sympathy-Lach, Natr. C., Nat. M., Nit. ac., Phos.

    (3) Desires cold food-Nat m., Phos.

    (4) Cold patient-Phos.

On 22-8-67 Phos. 200 was transmitted. Pain in tumor vanished at once and he felt much better. He was also given sac. lac. for one month.

On 15-9-67 tumor diminished in size and two abcesses formed near it, oozing out pus. The patient was nervous at this cathartic action. He was consoled and given sac. lac for one month more.

On 28-10-67, the abcesses had dried up and the size of tumor had reduced to 25%. The patient was advised to get Phos. 1M transmitted but instead he took it orally.

On 12-12-67 when the patient appeared, there was no trace of the tumor. He is in good health since then.

Case No. 11
Cancer Breast

On 22-2-70 Smt. K. of Champaran District, aged 39 years, came to the author for treatment of her troubles as mentioned below :-

(1)   She had painful lumps in breast-3 lumps in left and 2 in right. These were continuing for the last 6 months.

(2)   Bloody haemorrhoids since 1963.

(3)   Pain and burning in head since a long time.

(4)   Irregular menstruation.

She had suffered in the childhood from faintness and eczema. Her husband had miasms of syphilis and Sycosis.

Mind- (1) Weeping on listening to music.

(2) Sensation as if some living being was moving in abdomen.

(3) Despair. No point worth mentioning as far as desires and aversions are concerned. She was vegetarian.

(4) Stool-constipated, dry like balls.

(5) Dreams-dead body and falling.

Her remedy was selected on the following rubrics on the basis of Kent's repertory :-

(1)   Weeping on hearing music-Digi, Graph., Kreos., Kali. nit, Nat. C., Nat.S., Nux. Vom., Thuja.

(2)   Sensation as if living being were moving in abdomen-Nux-Vom.,Thuja.

(3)   Dreams of dead bodies-Thuja.

Thuja 200 was transmitted and Placebo was given for taking morning and evening.

On 28.2.70 she appeared and reported that she was menstruating since 24.2.70. Hence the transmission of Thuja was stopped.

On 2.4.70 she reported that the lumps had become soft. Carcin. 200 was transmitted.

On 23.4.70 she reported that menses had started on 4.4.70 and continued till 22.4.70. Transmission of carcinosin was continued.

On 17.5.70 it was found that the lumps were smaller. Thuja 0/6 was transmitted and Placebo was given.

On 3.6.70 the lumps were further reduced and pain too had decreased. Detaching from Thuja 0/6, Thuja 0/20 was transmitted and Placebo was given.

Afterwards Thuja 10M, Medorrh. C.M. Phytolacca 1M, Puls. 200 and 1M, Lycopodium 200 and 1M, Silicea 200, Carcinosin 1M, 10M were transmitted from time to time according to symptoms till 25.9.74.

She got rid of all her troubles and is having good health.

Case No. 12
Goiteric Cancer

Smt. Singh aged 54 of-Nawdah, Bihar had a tumor in the right side of external throat since one year but painful since 3 months. She had a small painful lymph gland near right ear also. She was examined by an Allopath who suspected it to be a case of cancer. Biopsy was advised. The Biopsy report declared it to be a case of "Goiteric Cancer" and 21.9.73 was fixed for operation. The patient had already seen the consequence (death) after operation of a cancer case in her neighbourhood hence she was afraid of undergoing it. She was advised by some gentlemen to consult the author hence she was brought to the author on 14.10.73 for treatment.

The following troubles and symptoms were noted-

(1)   The pain in her tumor (growth) was ameliorated by warmth and aggravated by cold exposure.

(2)   Pain in her right ear and throat was aggravated by empty swallowing.

(3)   There was tension in her whole throat since 3 months.

(4)   She had lumbago.

(5)   She had slight cough.

(6)   She had aversion to fat food and winter.

(7)   He weight was 40 Kg. only.

In her personal previous history as well as in her parents side there was nothing to mention. Her husband had been a victim of epilepsy in his young age. Husband's niece, and her eldest son had been victims of T.B. Her second son has been suffering from leucoderma. There was paucity of guiding symptoms. She had been under the treatment of an Allopath hence a routine Nux. Vom. 0/5 was transmitted through her hair and sufficient S.L. was given for a month on 14.10.73.

11.11.73-From 19.10.73 to 22.10.73 she had fever with headache. No improvement was noticed hence the previous transmission was made off and Calc. Fluor 1M was transmitted.

9.12.73-Her weight reduced by 2 Kg. No improvement. The weight was recorded as 38Kg. on 20.11.73.

The previous transmission was discontinued and Carcin. 35 was transmitted and sufficient S.L. was given. This transmission had a wonderful effect. Pain began to subside and weight started increasing with reduction of tumor in size.

13.1.74-Improving. Transmission continued after one plus (Throwing content of the phial and adding fresh dist. water with 10 strokes).

10.2.74-There was swelling on face and pain for 4 days. Transmission from the previous set was made off and Carcin. 200 was transmitted with sufficient S.L.

6.3.74-No trouble. Weight 48.5 Kg. the same transmission continued.

12.3.74-Transmission was continued after one plus and sufficient S.L. for a month.

29.4.74-   (1) Vertigo with nausea.

(2) Headache.

(3) Vertigo aggravated on rising from seat and motion.

Transmission was continued with another plussing.

2.6.74- (1) Tumor completely disappeared. No trace of it even on touch but there was sensation as if there were something in the right side of throat.

(2) Weight-49 Kg.

(3) Itching without eruptions.

(4) Pain in both knees which is aggravated while sitting and on rising from seat but ameliorated by motion.

(5) Thirst intense.

(6) No lumbago.

One more plus and then transmitted

7.7.74 - (1) Pain from neck to back.

(2) Sometimes headache aggravated by stooping and better by washing.

(3) Boil and sore on 1 foot and 1 thumb.

The transmission was discontinued and S.L. was transmitted in the above manner and S.L. was given to take morning and evening.

12.8.74 - (1) Weight 50 Kg.

(2) No trouble in back and neck.

(3) Feeling inconvenience in throat with cold. Carcin., 1 M. was transmitted and sufficient S.L. to take morning and evening.

16.9.74 - (1) From 2.9.74 difficulty in swallowing with tension in external throat but no growth of any kind. She looked anxious as sometimes the ghost of cancer hounded. No change in weight. After one plus Carcin. 1 M was transmitted.

12.10.74 - (1) Vertigo while lying as if the whole house was whirling since 4.10.74.

(2) Pain in throat on swallowing.

(3) Feeling heat.

(4) Fever from 20.9.74 to 24.9.74.

(5) Weight 49 Kg.

The transmission was made off and S.L. was transmitted and it was given for oral use for satisfaction.

15.11.74 - No trouble. Weight 50 Kg. Carcin. 1 M after further plussing was transmitted and sufficient S.L. was given to take morning and evening.

31.3.75 - The patient became irregular in treatment now and whenever she had some trouble in throat, she got frightened and then she came with throat trouble. Pain in throat on swallowing which was ameliorated by external warmth and warm dink.

The transmission was made off and S.L. was transmitted. Sufficient S.L. given to take orally morning and evening.

2.5.75 -   (1) Neck pain.

(2) Right sided headache occasionally from 15.4.75.

(3) Eczema reappeared in 1 finger of hand since 1.4.75.

(4) Mouth dry.

(5) Weight 51 Kg.

No change in medicine. S.L. was transmitted and given for oral use.

22.5.75 - She did not turn up and it was learnt from messenger that she had no trouble now. Hence treatment was discontinued. She is quite hale and hearty. The ghost does not haunt her. She is completely free from the malignant growth.

Case No. 13
Gums Cancer

Sri Singh, aged 36 years, Headmaster of a Middle School in Patna district had been suffering from gums Cancer since 1975. There was a growth around the caried molar in the left upper gums which was extracted in March, 1974. Biopsy report on 10.4.75 revealed :

"Microscopic Stratified squamous epithelial cells seen. At places strands of squamous epithelial cells seen penetrating the deeper tissue. These cells show hypercromatic appearance of the nuclei".

Diagnosis-"Squamous cell carcinoma".

Left lower gum was ulcerated and there was pus discharge with pain since 10.4.75. He was advised to undergo cobalt therapy and 18 exposures were given till 14.5.75. He was feeling much relief till 17.8.75. But trouble started since 18.8.75 hence he was brought to the author on 23.8.75.

The following troubles were noted-

1. Right upper gum was swollen and painful with a small growth around the caried molar since 19.8.75.
2. Pus was coming out from his right ear since 18.8.75.
3. Edges of tongue were ulcerated.
4. Pain in right ear and temple.
5. Boils on the left hip and thigh since a month.
6. Appetite less after cobalt therapy.
7. A rough small wart on his right forearm since one month.
8. Loss of weight.
9. Inner side of cheeks were peeling off.

Previous troubles-

1. Caries in 3 molars.
2. Ringworm and itches 68.
3. Otorrhoea in left ear in 1971.
4. Crablice and body lice.
5. Haematuria in 1962.
6. Injury to eyebrow in 1973-profuse bleeding.
7. Urticaria 16 years back.
8. Cramping pain in legs.
9. Falling of hair in beard.

Father aged 60 had been a victim of syphilis and suspected T.B.

Mother has been suffering from asthma.

Grand mother had been a patient of asthma. His maternal uncle has anaesthetic skin.

One cousin had T.B. and Epilepsy.

Another cousin died of cancer in sole in 1974. One uncle died of Haemorhoids and Cancer in rectum.

He was married in 1960 and his wife has caried teeth.

His first son died after birth at night. He has 4 sons and 4 daughters suffering from otorrhoea.

Mind-He is a fatalist but had suicidal tendency in April 1974, by poison or cutting. He used to weep to see friends and relatives. Weeping was aggravated by consolation.

He is hopeful of recovery.

Head-Dandruff and lice

Likes-Meat and sweets.

He used to sleep covering his mouth and nose even in summer with dreams of dead person.

Pain in ear, temple and gums was aggravated in night and ameliorated by lying on painful side and warmth.

23.8.75-   Cobalt 30 was transmitted and sufficient S.L. was given to take one globule morning and evening.

3.9.75-   1.   Burning in inner cheeks. Left eye pain aggravated in evening.

            2.   Abscess of hip healed up.

            3.   Good appetite.

            4.   Tingling in feet on rising in morning.

            5.   No tears on seeing people.

            6.   Weight 59 Kg.

14.9.75 -   1.   Pain aggravated by cold water.

            2.   One style on eyelid right side since 10.9.75.

            3.   Cramping pain in legs since 12.9.75.

            4.   Teeth sensitive as if sand under.

            5.   Weight 59 Kg.

Hair was detached from cobalt 30 solution and Carcin.

1M was transmitted with S.L. to be continued.

22.9.75 -   1.   Otorrhoea-thick pus continued.

            2.   Stye on eyelid vanished.

            3.   Cramping pain in legs also vanished.

            4.   White coated tongue.

            5.   Desire for salty things.

            6.   Weight 60 Kg.

No change in medicine simply one plus was done with 10 strokes.

3.10.75 - Toothache agg by cold application. Again one plus and it vanished like magic.

24.10.75 - (1) White-coated tongue,

2) Swelling on cheek,

(3) Saliva in mouth,

(4) Weight 59.5 Kg. One plus.

13.11.75 - (1) Swelling in left cheek and eye, with burning.

(2) Saliva less,

(3) Itching in body,

(4) Weight 61 Kg.

(5) Wart on forearm disappeared.

One more plus with 10 strokes and S.L.

17.12.75 - Pain in left eye aggravated from 28.11.75.

6th plus with 10 strokes and S.L.

31.12.75 - (1) Weight 60 Kg.

(2) Pain in left eye and left inner cheek aggravated by cold and ameliorated by warmth,

(3) Falling of hair in left side beard,

(4) Lousiness.

Hair was detached from Carcin. 1M and S.L. was dissolved and transmitted. S.L. was given to be continued.

31.1.76 - (1) Weight 61 Kg.

(2) Swelling with pain in right upper gums from 23.1.76 to 25.1.76 only,

(3) Seminal discharge with urine,

(4) Ringworm in the left side chest without itching from 15.1.76,

(5) Pain in left arm when raising since 31.1.76,

(6) White coated tongue.

One plus in this S.L. Solution also.

14.2.76 - (1) Ringworm on chest disappeared,

(2) Body lice,

(3) Bloody pus form right ear,

(4) Weight 60 Kg.

(5) Growth of gum vanished.

Carcin 1 M was made 8 pluses with 10 strokes each time and then transmitted, with S.L. to continue.

1.3.76 - (1) Abscess in right ankle, from 27.2.76 due to shoe pinch-bleeding and abscess broke open on 29.2.76,

(2) Flatulence.

(3) Itching upper lip from 29.2.76,

(4) Cold and cough,

(5) Weight 60.5 Kg.

Transmission was put off and now All. Cep. 30 was transmitted to cover shoe pinch.

22.3.76 - 1. Weakness and feverish since 18.3.76.

2. Tingling from hands and feet vanished since 18.3.76.

3. Headache and ear pain since 20.3.76.

4. One abscess in right thigh since 12.3.76.

5. Weight 60.5 Kg.

M.S. 200 was transmitted.

19.5.76 - Abscesses from right thigh, hip and left leg vanished.

2. Bloody discharge from ear continued.

3. White coated tongue.

4. Urticaria from 4.5.76.

5. Weight 61 Kg.

Detached from 200 and M.S. 1 M was transmitted.

29.5.76 - 1. Weight 61 Kg.

2. Head Heavy.

One plus with 10 strokes.

24.7.76 - 1. Pain in gums,

2. Left eye heavy,

3. Weight 62.5 Kg.

5 Pluses and S.L.

20.10.76 - 1. Fever on 29-30 September, 76.

           2. Fever blisters,

           3. Crablice.

           4. No otorrhoea since 1.10.76.

           5. Itches in legs.

           6. Cold and cough from 1.10.76.

           7. Weight 61 Kg.

           8. No ulceration and pain etc. in mouth.

Detached from M.S. 1 M and Sabad. 1 M was transmitted.

15.11.76 - No trouble. Hard labour : he used to go to school and back on cycle 20 miles per day, Transmission continued.

19.1.77 - (1) Weight 59 Kg.

           (2) Diarrhoea since 14.1.77.

           (3) Pain in gums with swelling.

           (4) Lice and crablice persist,

           (5) Right side neck painful.

Sypm. 10 M-transmitted with S.L.

13.3.77 - No troubles. Weight 60.5 Kg. Going on quite well but labours hard as usual.

According to new project i.e. a series of potencies at a time-Syph. 10 M and C.M. were transmitted separately in three phials.

15.4.77 - (1) Weight 62 Kg.

           (2) No trouble

Continued with one plus each.

10.5.77 - No trouble. Continued with one plus more. He is doing hard work still he is leading a normal life. Ghost of cancer does not hover his mind.

12.6.77 - Weight 64.5 Kg., Quite Well.

Case No. 14

Throat Cancer

Sri Singh aged 45 of Sitamarhi, Bihar had been suffering from throat cancer as the Biopsy report revealed. There was a round growth located in the right side effecting the right side of the post part of the tongue since December, 1973. He had been under the modern treatment and had 16 exposures of deep X-Ray by the end of March, 1974. Even after the so called wonderful therapy, there was a smooth firm growth in the throat which had been giving much trouble from time to time. He was treated by a renowned Homoepath of Gorakhpur in April 1975 but without any relief.

The patient has no knowledge of this disease hence ignorance is a bliss in this case. He was brought to the author on 10.8.75 with the following complaints-

(1)   The mouth was very dry after X-Ray Therapy.

(2)   The throat was full of phlegm, feeling difficulty in breathing and swallowing.

(3)   Had hoarseness of voice.

(4)   Tongue scalded and swollen.

(5)   Heart burning.

(6)   Ring-worm since 20 year.

(7)   Sciatica, lift side, for the last 6 years.

(8)   Appetite decreased much since 2 ½ months.

(9)   Swelling of face right side since 1 ½ months.

Previous troubles -

(1)   T.B. 6 years ago treated by Allopaths.

(2)   Malaria and use of Quinine long ago.

(3)   Snake-bite.

(4)   Abscess in the right axilla-8 months back operated.

(5)   Had history of scabies, measles and vaccinations.

(6)   Wrestling from 18 to 38 years age.

Parents died in old age. One of his uncles died of T.B. 5 years back. His eldest brother has high blood-pressure and Leucoderma.

Mind -   Fear of thunderstorm.

Sympathetic by nature.

Craving for salty things. Sciatica pain aggravated by east wind and sitting for a while but ameliorated by motion, lying on painful side and pressure.

10.8.75 -   To antidote the effect of X-Ray, X-Ray 200 was transmitted.

17.8.75 -   Hair was detached from X-Ray and Carcin. 200 was transmitted.

24.8.75 -   Carcin. was detached due to severe headache, body pain, weakness and dysentery, Nux. vom. 0/3 was transmitted.

11.12.75 - There was increase in swelling of tongue, preventing swallowing and breathing. Loss of appetite and weakness for 10 days. Nux. Vom was detached and Carb. Veg. 1 M was transmitted. He passed two big roundworms and many thread worms on the 12th and 13th January 76.

3.2.76 -   Hair was detached form C.V. 1 M solution as there was severe throat pain. Placebo was transmitted.

21.4.76 -   N. V. 200 was transmitted when there was a very painful swelling of tongue with breathing difficulty and fever.

1.6.77 -   Transmission of N.V. was put off because of a swelling and pain in left cheek and a lump therein.

Cervical region was also painful and tongue very dry.

The case was repertorised as follows vide Kent's Repertory -

1.   Sympathy - Carl., Caust., Cic., Croc., Ig., Iod., Lyc., Manc., N.C., N.M., N.A., Nuph., N.V., Phos, and Puls.

2.   Fear thunderstorm - N.C.,N.M., N.A., Phos.

3.   Craving for meat - N.M.

N.M.200 was transmitted.

24.7.76 -   No complaints.

N.M. 1 M.-Transmitted.

11.8.76 -   Condition better - simply plussing it.

9.9.76 -   Do

18.10.76 - Hair was detached form N.M. 1 M due to pain in right ear with discharge and fever. Heart burning aggravated in the afternoon.

Desire for salt decreased.

Sepia 200 was transmitted.

31.10.76 - No pus. Pain in ear from 19.10.76 to 23.10.76. One tumor appeared in the right cheek with swelling of right temple with pain etc. Hair was detached from Sepia 200 and Placebo was transmitted. The tumor suppurated, broke open and healed up by 30.10.76.

16.11.76 - Thick and yellow discharge from the right ear and pain better by cold application. Puls. 200 was transmitted.

24.12.76 - Pus continued. 2 Pluses.

19.4.77 - Pus continued but better in all respects, N.M. 10 M was transmitted.

17.5.77 - Fever from 5.5.77, detached and fever stopped form 17.5.77.

The patient came on 18.5.77 with slight pain in back and neck, aggravated by sitting and motion. That too vanished by 18.5.77. Due to continued fever he lost two Kg. in weight. The treatment was continued by correspondence and he used to come the author after long intervals. He is gaining weight and there is no sign of growth either in the throat or in the cheeks. He has no trouble now but the care will be followed up for years.

Case No. 15
Throat Cancer

Shri Hardeo Dubey, aged 55 years, office peon of Cane Inspector, Shri B.N. Shrama of Bettiah had a cancerous growth in the left side of his throat, and parotid gland was very much enlarged. He was diagnosed at Patna Medical College and Hospital and was given radium treatment, but to no effect. The growth was rapid, voice affected and was unable to swallow even water. The doctors had given up all hopes of his life and so he consulted the author on 17.10.68. Lachesis 2 C was transmitted with immediate relief of throat pain and he was able to take solid and liquid. However, there was no marked reduction in the growth. Carcinosin 2 C was transmitted on 22.11.68 and Lachesis was transmitted on 22.12.68. On 26.1.69 it was noticed that the entire growth of the throat had vanished and he was trouble-free. But the size of the parotid gland was reduced by 50% only and hence Lachesis 10 M was transmitted on 9.3.69 with the result that the remaining growth of parotid gland also vanished.

During treatment he gained 5 lbs. of weight too. Once he g t some respiratory trouble which could not be controlled like magic hence he changed treatment.

Case No. 16

Uterine Cancer

Smt. S.R. Devi aged. 48 of Bikramganj, Rohtas had been suffering from metrorrhagia from September, 1973. Biopsy test declared it on 26.11.73 to be a case of Cancer. (Squamous cell carcinoma State III) in Cervix. There was a Cauliflower like growth in the Cervix. The Cancer Specialist advised to undergo Cobalt Therapy. Hence she had exposures of Cobalt for a month in December, 1973. She had without acute trouble for about a year but had weakness. Metastasis started and the rectum was involved by a malignant growth. She had haemorrhage from rectum from February, 1975. She could not go for Radium therapy and was brought to the author on 17.8.75. She suffered from the ailments mentioned below :-

(1)   Bleeding from rectum with stool and while passing flatus past six months.

(2)   2-4 loose stools (daily) for the last six months.

(3)   Dry Eczema since 2 years.

(4)   Hard of hearing after loss of blood from uterus.

(5)   Lumbago from September, 1973.

(6)   Filarial swelling in right leg since last 10 days.

Weight :- 45 Kilograms :-

Earlier personal ailments

(i)   Suffered from Small Pox at 12 years of age.

(ii)   Fracture in left knee in 1972.

(iii) Shoulder pain on right side.

Parents had good longivity. Three sisters and one brother are almost normal.

She was married in 1942. Her husband has leucoderma on his lip. His father had been a victim of Gonorrhoea and Asthma. Patient's four sons and three daughters are alive and healthy. Her first son died one month after birth and she had one abortion.

Mental Symptoms :-

    (1)   Sympathetic by nature.

    (2)   Fear of darkness.

    (3)   Weeps for not being able to see her kith and kin, consolation aggravates.

    (4)   Weeps while narrating her troubles.

    (5)   Becomes sad on hearing music and

    (6)   She doubted her recovery.

Head — Headache on speaking and weeping, dandruff.

Likes — Fish, meat, chillies and sour things.

Dislikes— Milk and fat.

Stool — Is driven out of bed for stool at 4 a.m. Gripping pain in lower abdomen before stool. Hard Tumour in anus and haemorrhage during stool.

Sleep — Disturbance in sleep due to anxiety. Lying on left side gave comfort. Dreams of snake-bite.

Lumbago—Better lying on back.

Lower extremities :- Filarial swelling on right leg.

Sensation :- Coldness in lower abdomen.

Generalities :- Better in winter season.

    Worse standing and in the sun.

    The case was repertorised with help of Kent's Repertory and Kishore's Card in the following way :-

(1)   Dislikes fat (Ghee):- Ang., Ars. Alb., Bell., Bry., C.C., Carb an., Carb. S., C.V., China., Chin. A., Colch., Croc., Cycl., Dros., Grat., Guare., Hell., Hep., lyss., Meny., M.S., Nat. a., N.C., N.M., Petr., Phos., Ptel., Puls., Rheum., R.T., Sang., Sec., Sep. and Sulph.

(2)   Dislikes Milk :- Ars. Alb., Bell., Bry., C.C., Carb. an., Cycl., Hep., M.S., N.C., N.M., Phos., Puls., R.T., Sec., Sep. and Sulph.

(3)   Sympathetic :- N.C., N.M., Puls. and Phos.

(4)   Consolation aggr. : - N.M. and Sepia.

(5)   Desires :- Fish - N.M.

Nat. Mur. runs through all the above rubrics hence it seemed to be a similimum.

17.8.75 :- Nat. Mur. 0/3 (one globule of no. 10) was dissolved into a dram phial containing distilled water and 10 strokes were given to the phial. No sooner her hair was inserted into that phial. She began to feel cheerful and fresh. Her palms became warm and began sweating. Sensation of coldness on abdomen vanished like magic. Sufficient S.L. was given to be taken one globule morning and evening.

21.9.75 :- Profuse bleeding from anus on 18.9.75 at 8 A.M. after passing of flatus.

The hair was detached from N.M. and Phos. 0/6 was transmitted in a similar manner. Just after this transmission, there was rumbling sound in her abdomen and sensation of coldness on abdomen reappeared.

19.10.75:- (1) She experienced vertigo and colic on 29.9.75.

(2) Bleeding from anus on 2nd and 3rd October, 1975.

(3) Itching without any eruption.

(4) Aggravation in the swelling of the leg.

Detaching hair from Phos., Sepia 200 was transmitted and S.L.

16.11.75 - No trouble but pain in foot due to injury. After one plus with 10 strokes Sepia was retransmitted and S.L.

14.12.75 - (1) Bleeding from anus for 6 days.

(2) Pain in right shoulder.

(3) Fever blisters on left corner of lower lip, and

(4) Feeling feverish.

Again after one plus transmission was continued and S.L.

21.1.76 - (1) Profuse bleeding from anus.

(2) Toothache.

(3) Pain of right shoulder disappeared.

N.V. 200 was transmitted after detaching from Sepia 200 and S.L.

29.2.76 - (1) Weight 44.5 Kg. and

(2) Bleeding for seven days.

Detaching from N.V. Carcin. 200 was transmitted and

S.L.

28.3.76 -   (1) Very less bleeding, clotted and dark blood.

(2) No other troubles.

After three pluses carcin. 200 was again transmitted.

2.5.76 - Aggrav. in swelling of leg.

Detaching from the previous medicine, N.M. 1000 was transmitted.

6.6.76 -   (1) Weight 46 Kg. and

(2) No troubles.

One plus in N.M. 1000 and S.L.

10.7.76 -   (1) Acute pain in right knee since 8.7.76.

(2) Fever on 9.7.76.

(3) Very less bleeding.

(4) Lumbago acute since to-day.

(5) Weight 44.5 Kg.

Detached from N.M., Arnica 200 was transmitted to relieve pain as she had fallen against back on 25.6.76 but to no effect. Detaching from Arnica, R.T. 200 was transmitted. Pain vanished like magic.

15.8.76 -   (1) Very scanty bleeding.

(2) Good health and weight 45 Kg.

(3) Good sleep.

(4) No lumbago or knee pain.

(5) Itching in Eczema relieved by cold application.

Detaching from R.T., Puls 200 was transmitted and S.L.

10.10.76 -   (1) Fever from 3.10.76.

(2) Fever blisters on lips.

(3) Tongue aphthous.

(4) Itching in Eczema aggravated by cold application.

(5) Weight 45.5 Kg.

Detached from puls 200, Sepia 200 after two pluses was transmitted.

5.12.76 -   (1) No bleeding.

(2) Injury to left leg.

(3) Pain in leg aggravated in beginning of motion but relieved by motion.

(4) Weight 45 Kg.

Detaching from Puls 200, R.T. 200 after two pluses was transmitted. Pain relieved at once.

25.12.76 - (1) Fever with shivering on 23.12.76.

(2) Pain in whole body.

(3) Involuntary urination while passing flatus on 24th and 25th Dec. 76.

The previous transmission was put off and Sepia IM was transmitted.

30.12.76 - (1) Fever 101⁰.

(2) Profuse bleeding.

(3) Severe attack of filaria.

(4) Injury after falling down.

Detaching from Sepia Arnica 200 was transmitted.

29.11.77 - (1) Bleeding only on 24.1.77.

(2) Fever with shivering (old symptom).

Carcin. 200 after one plus was transmitted.

12.3.77 - (1) Very scanty blood from anus.

(2) Swelling of leg persisting.

(3) Bleeding after scratching.

(4) Aversion to fats.

(5) Weight 45.5 Kg.

Note - One project to shorten the duration of cure has been taken up by the Research Institute of Sahni Drug Transmission and Homoeopathy, by transmitting a series of potencies of the selected drug at a time in different phials. Hence according to this project, Puls IM, 10 M, 50 M and C.M. in 4 different phials were transmitted through 4 hairs of the patient.

24.4.77 - (1) No trouble.

(2) Eczema and swelling of leg still continues.

(3) very good health.

(4) No anxiety.

(5) Sound sleep.

(6) Tumour of anus disappeared.

One plus of each set and S.L.

27.5.77 -   (1) Very good health without troubles.

(2) Swelling and Eczema very much decreased.

(3) Ghost of Cancer no more.

(4) Weight 46 Kg.

Transmission is continued to follow the case up.

Case No. 17
Uterine Cancer

Mrs. G. Debi aged 65 of Gaya, had been suffering from uterine cancer. On 2-9-1976 Biopsy was done which was declared to be "Squamous cell carcinoma grade two" Just after it was declared to be fatal, her son brought her to the author on 9.9.1970 for her treatment.

The case was taken up earnestly and the following symptoms were taken for selection of similimum :-

1.   She had been suffering from bloody and offensive leucorrhoea since one year.

2.   She had metrorrhagia since six months.

3.   Her husband had been a victim to syphilis and out of 9 children only 8 were alive.

4.   She was given to uttering abuses.

5.   She had the habit of cursing.

.   She was Jealous by nature.

7.   She had craving for (ghee) fat.

The case was repertorised by Kent. Repertory in the following manner :-

1.   Cursing - Aloe, Am, c., Anac., Ars., Bell., Bor., Boy., Cann.,i., Cauth., Cor. r., Gal. ac., Hycs., Ip., Lac. c., Lil. tig., Lyc., Lyss., Nat. m., Nit ac. Nux vom., Oena., Op., Pall., Petr., Plb., Puls., Stra., Tub., Verat.

2.   Abusive - Am.c., Anc., Bell., Bor., Hyas., Ip. B. Byc., N. ac., N.V., Petr., Plb, Stram., Tub., Verat.

3.   Syphilis - N.ac.Petr.

4.   Desires - Fat (ghee)- N. ac.

9.9.1970 - Only N.ac. runs through all the above rubrics hence
it was selected as similimum and transmitted in the
200th potency. Sufficient S.L. was given for a month
to be taken morning and evening. She was advised
to report weekly about her weight. She went away
to Purnea from Patna.

10.10.1970-After transmission, foul smell of Leucorrhoea began
to decrease and after a week from the date of
transmission (9.9.70) Leucorrrhoea and blood
discharge ceased completely. Her husband breathed
his last on 24.9.70, which was like a blow from the
blue to her. She was mentally upset and, watery
discharges from her vagina began. Transmission of
N.A. was discontinued and Ign 200 was transmitted.

25.10.70 - Report through a messanger-Discharge having for
some days continued from 19.10.70 to 24.10.70.
Transmission of Ign. was discontinued and N.A. 200
after plussing (one globule diluted into one dram
phial Containing distilled water and throwing all
the contents of that phial till about one drop is left
in the phial and it was filled again with distilled
water and given 10 strokes. This is formed one plus
by the author was transmitted. S.L. was given to be
continued.

6.11.70 - From 26.10.70 discharge decreased till 1.11.70 and
from 2.11.70 stopped completely.

12.12.70 - (1) Slight bleeding came 24.11.70, 30.11.70, 7.12.70
and 12.12.70.

(2) Appetite good

(3) Sometimes foul leucorrhoea.

Carcinosin 200 was transmitted and sufficient S.L. was
given. Weight was not noted inspite of repeated reminders.
Again she was advised to get herself weighed.

19.1.1971 - Slight bleeding on 1.1.71 and 15.1.71. Her weight on
12.1.71 was 48 Kg. N.A. IM was transmitted and
sufficient S.L. was given to be taken

19.2.71 - Bleeding on 28.1.71 and offensive leucorrhoea from
29.1.71 weight 49 Kg. N.A. IM was transmitted
after one plussing.

23.3.71 - (1) no change in weight.

(2) Slight blood discharge on 20.2.71 and slight leucorrhoea N.ac. IM Transmission was discontinued and carcinosin 200 was transmitted after one plussing.

2.4.71 - Weight on 30.3.71 - 48 Kg. Carcin 200 transmission was continued and the transmitting set was handed over to the messenger with an instruction to discontinue the present transmission in case she loses her weight and bleeding starts. S.L. was diluted in one dram phial and given to insert hair into that S.L. containing solution after detaching hair from carcinosin 200. Sufficient S.L. for oral use was given.

20.4.71- Weight 49.5 Kg. No trouble.

27.4.71- Weight 50 Kg. No trouble treatment was discontinued inspite of repeated advice to continue it at least for 2 years. She assumed her to be perfectly cured. Still the case was followed at for 2 years and she had no trouble.

Note :- 1. The patient came to the author at Patna twice only and she remained at Purnea with her son during treatment. From second month of treatment. She began to say that she was cured. She is an innocent lady having no knowledge of prognosis of the malignant disease but her son knowing fully well, persuaded her to continue so far.

2. Generally the transmitting set means-one dram phial containing solution of one globule of the selected remedy in distilled water and one end of one hair of the patient inserted into that solution and another end floating in air.

3. The transmitting set was kept at Patna and the patient was getting its radiation at Purnea.

Case No. 18
Cancer of Uterus

On 16.9.72 Smt. K. Kumari of Muz. aged 35 years, came to the author for treatment. She had the following troubles :

(a) She was suffering from irregular and copious menstruation with leucorrhoea for the last 14 years.

(b) For some time she had low fever aggr. from 12 noon to 9 P.M.

(c) Lumbago for the last 10 years.

(d) All the troubles were on left side of her body.

(e) Constipation.

(f) Had pain in chest for 2 years and one small wart on right cheek. It was a declared case of uterine cancer.

Previous troubles :

(a) Malaria at 10 years age which was treated with quinine.

(b) Had pus formation in vagina and swelling in 1953.

(c) Birth of a dead child.

In family history, her husband had suffered from syphilis and gonorrhoea 14 years back. She as married in 1954,

The following points were taken into account in selection of remedy :

(a) Weeping after anger and when listening to music.

(b) Worse after eating.

(c) Nature-Sympathetic, obstinate and revengeful.

(d) Tendency to commit suicide.

(e) Desires-Milk and Ghee, warm food.

She had been under allopathic treatment for a pretty long time.

On 16.9.92, Nux. Vom. 200 was transmitted. As a result the haemorrhage stopped from 25.9.72. After one month the same remedy was transmitted after plussing.

From 14.11.72 as her taste changed and she began to like cold food and the miasms of Syphilis and Sycosis had to be antidoted, hair was detached form N.V. and Thuja 200 was transmitted. This gave good results and improvement in health set in.

On 24.3.73 - Menstruation became regular and normal but leucorrhoea persisted. This same remedy was transmitted after plussing.

On 9.6.73 - General health better, but occasionally she had discharges. Detached from Thuja 200 and transmitted Thuja IM.

On 7.10.73 - She had been feeling free from all troubles except some pain in lumber region. Detached from Thuja IM and transmitted Rhus. Tox. 200. The lumber pain vanished immediately.

On 4.4.74 - She again complained of pain in the left extremities and hypogastrium. There was neither menstrual trouble nor leucorrhoea. General health was good. Detached from Rhus. Tox. and transmitted Thuja 10M. She was free from her troubles by April, 74.

She is still enjoying a good health.

Case No. 19
Colic

Shri B. Mistry aged 45 of Bhagalpur was chronic patient of peptic ulcer. Her was operated upon but after a year his trouble got back. He was under the treatment of the Late Dr. R.C. Shastry. He was one day in great agony and his doctor was out of the station. Seeing the effect of transmission on other patients he came to the author on 4.4.67 only for some relief. His symptoms were noted in short. He had a severe pain in his right hypochondrium shooting to his right scapula. The taste of his mouth was bitter. He liked hot food and drinks. His pain was relieved temporarily after eating. Pressure on the painful part also gave him relief. Chelidon. 6 was transmitted and his pain was reduced at once and he slept in the chamber for hours. Then he woke up and went home being free from his pain that day. Next day he came to the author but he was directed to go to his doctor. Unwillingly he obeyed him.

Case No. 20
Colic

Mrs, Mahamaya Kumari, aged 18 of village Lailak, Bhagalpur had severe colic in her umblical region which was aggravated by slight movement. Bell. 200 was transmitted. At once she felt giddy and put her head on the table. Then she left the table to go out but became blind for a moment. She vomited at 5.30 P.M. food taken at 11 A.M. just on the verandah as she could not go outside. After sometimes she had a clear stool also and slept for one hour. She became free from her trouble after waking.

Case No. 21
Colic

Master Devilal Choudhary aged 17 of Mandroja Mahalla, Bhagalpur, came to consult the author for his colic. Sulph. 200 one globule was brought in contact with one of his hair from his head at the distance of 8 feet. He was free from his colic instantaneously.

Case No. 22
Colic

Bulu's mother aged about 50 of Bhagalpur had been suffering from intense colic in her right illiac region for 4 days. It was diagnosed as acute appendicitis. Pain was aggravated by jerks and cold, and ameliorated by warm application. She was brought in a rickshaw which was horrible for her. Bell 200. One globule was transmitted through her hair at a distance of 10 .feet. Instantaneously she began to belch without a break for 5 minutes and then she was free from her colic like a magic.

Case No. 23
Colic

Mrs. K. Sinha, M.A. (Pol. Sc.) of Bettiah aged 28 had been suffering from intense colic pain in the liver region. Local Drs. of repute had diagnosed her to be suffering from Gall Bladder stone and had advised her operation by some eminent surgeon of the State. She had been to Patna for this purpose but as good luck would have it the operation could not be performed for some reasons or other. Ultimately she consulted the author on the 13th October, 1968 and she was diagnoised as Lachasis and 200th potency of it as transmitted to her with the result that she had never been attacked by her colic pain. Then after some months she conceived and delivered a healthy female child safely.

Case No. 24
Writer's Cramp

Shri K.N. Lal, aged 35, District Industry Officer, Gaya,

consulted the author on 16.4.1967 for his following troubles :-

(1)   Writer's cramp

(2)   Skin rough and scaly and

(3)   Tooth loose and painful.

Previous personal ailments :-

(1)   Kalazar

(2)   Itches treated externally

(3)   Measles and

(4)   Influenza.

Mind :-   Liking for loneliness. He was growing indifferent and irritable His irritation was highly aggravated by consolation.

Head :-   Dandruff aggravated in winter.

Mouth :-   Taste salty, normal thirst. Looseness of teeth with pain.

Likes :-   Sweets and hot food.

Dislikes :- Milk.

Extremities :- Fidgety in lower limbs and coldness in legs. Cramping in right hand when writing.

Skin :-   Rough and scaly. Worse in bends of elbows and knees.

Modalities :-   A chilly patient-worse winter and better summer. The case was repertorised by Kent's Repertory (Ist Indian Edition) as follows :-

Excluding hot remedies.

(1)   Dislikes milk :-

Am. C, Bell., Calc., C. V., Cina, Lac. d., Led., M.C., N.C., N.P., N. V., Phos., Sep., Sil., Stann.

(2)   Consolation aggravates - Bell, Calc., Sep., Sil. (Page 93)

(3)   Likes loneliness - Bell., Calc., Sep.   (Page 12)

(4)   Fidgety-Lower Limbs-Bell., Sep. (Page 1187)

(5)   Scaly skin - Bell., Sep. (Page 1319)

(6)   Suppression of Itches - Bell., Sep. (Page 1319)

(7)   Cramps in extremities - Bell, Sep. (Page 917)

(8)   Dandruff - Sep. (Page 114)

(9)   Looseness of teeth - Sep. (Page 433)

Sepia covers the totality of symptoms hence it was thought to be transmitted from Bhagalpur to Gaya at a distance of 228 K. M. One hair from his head was brought to Bhagalpur from where Sepia 10M was transmitted on 19.4.67. After a week it was reported that the medicine had no effect. On 1.5.67 one globule Sepia 50 M. was brought in contact with that hair. After a week it was reported that it had some effect.

(1) Less scales,   (2) No pain in teeth and looseness was also less (3) There was improvement in cramps also.   (4) He was feeling much better.

He was free from all troubles by the end of July 1967.

Case No. 25
Cyst

Sri....Sinha aged 42 an Officer of the Education Department, Bihar had a medium plumb sized Cyst on his Right wrist for the last two years. The case was taken up on 30.12.1973 on the initiative of the author himself. There was pausity of Symptoms hence on one rubric i.e. "Cyst on wrist" Cal. Carb was selected. Cal. Carb 0/3 was transmitted, which continued upto 6.9.74 without any charge in the Cyst. Then Lyco 1M was transmitted on 6.9.74 after detaching the hair from C.C. It also could not reduce the size of the Cyst, though there was some improvement in general health. The patient could not report hence transmission of Lyco 1M was continued till 3.12.74 Carcin 1M was transmitted after detaching hair from the previous Transmitting Set which remained continued for a long time. Perchance the author met Sri Sinha on 12.1.77 and found no trace of the Cyst on his wrist. On enquiry it was learnt that it had disappeared completely in June, 1976. Hence Transmission was set off finally.

Case No. 26
Dead Sperm Made Alive

Sri N. aged 40 had no issue though he was married at the age of 25. Seminal fluid examination reports for 12 years revealed that all sperms had died. The modern therapy could not help him. He came to the author for treatment on 15.4.1971.

He had the following troubles :-

(1)   All sperms dead.

(2)   Vericose Veins in both spermatic cords.

(3)   Susceptible to cold since childhood.

(4)   Flatulence since long.

(5)   Occasional body pain.

(6)   Dandruff in head.

Previous personal ailments :-

(1)   Measles long ago.

(2)   Onanism in young age.

(3)   Jaundice in 1967.

(4)   Tonsils were operated in 1967.

Mind :-   Pessimist, Introvert and shy by nature. Habit of nail biting with teeth. Full of planning. Sympathetic.

Likes :-   Vegetarian, nut and Salty things.

Dislikes :- Milk and Sweets.

Stomach :- Flatulence aggravated in evening and ameliorated by eating.

Stool :-   Thrice daily, but once just after lunch.

M.S. Org :- More sexual desire with quick discharge.

Sleep :-   Sound. Two pillows were being used for resting the head.

Extremities:-   Pain in calves while lying on bed in morning and night which was ameliorated by massage. Fidgity.

Worse :-   Evening and Standing.

Better :-   Summer and Coition.

The following rubrics were considered for selection of remedy.

(1)   Sympathy and shyness.

(2)   Likes salty things.

(3)   Dislikes milk and sweets.

(4)   Onanism.

Phos. scored highest.

Phos. 200 was transmitted on 16.4.71. Transmission was switched off on 20.4.71 because of fever and aggravation of pain in the extremities from 17.4.71, but spermatic cords felt loose and painful.

Hamamelis 30, Euphrasia 30,Ferr. Met. 200 were transmitted from time to time according to change of symptoms. Seminal fluid was examined on 9.8.1971. and the following report was given :-

Total number of sperms-44000000

Motality after ejaculation 60% actively motile.

Motality one hour after 56%

Motality 2 hours after 48%

Motality 6 hours after 29%

21% abnormal.

The treatment was continued by transmitting Ferr. Met IM, China 30,200 Lyco IM 0/3, 0/5 from time to time till 1.4.73. It was discontinued due to his transfer from Patna. In the meantime his wife conceived and gave birth to a female child but unfortunately the baby died.

Case No. 27
Diabetes

Sri V. of Monghyr aged 48 who had been suffering from Diabetes since 1966, Came to the author for Treatment on 3.9.1973, He had the following troubles:-

(1)   Diabetes for 7 years.

(2)   Tingling in left leg for 2 years.

(3)   Pain in lower extremities for 1 year.

(4)   Constipation

(5)   Urinary Trouble.

Past Personal Ailments:-

(1)   Injury to right leg in childhood.

(2)   Syphilis at the age of 18 years.

(3)   Skin disease suppressed by ext. application.

(4)   Vasectomy 7 years back.

(5)   Hydrocele left side, operated 7 Years back.

Father alive-Diabetes and anaesthesia.

Mother died of T.B. when the patient was 5 years old.

Step mother died of Diabetes.

His sister's husband died of T.B.

He was married 32 years back and his wife had various ailments. He was seven sons and one daughter. Almost all suffered from cold and cough and Tonsilities. One son suffered from rheumatism two Sons have stammering, one has lipoma and another son has been suffering from asthmatic trouble.

Mind :-   Abusive, Anger increased, Fear downward motion and noises, nervous temperament, Indicisive, Hopeful, Cosmopoliton by nature, weeping in anger, prayer and sympathy and memory weak for recent events.

Li .king for Fat, Ghee and Milk.

Aversion to non-vegetarian Food.

Stomach :- Slow digestion, better before eating, Eructation Nausea while brushing in the morning and constipation-used to go to latrine 3 or 4 times daily.

Urine :-   Sugar, burning in urethra, Interrupted and hurry to pass.

M.Sex. Org :-   Desire diminished, incomplete erection and quick discharge.

Sleep :-   Sound, on left side with high pillow.

Dreams :-   Amorous, Journey, feast, Urine etc.

Tingling and Pain in lower extremities aggravated by motion and in night.

Better :-   Summer.

Worse :-   In Extremes of climate, bad news, noises.

The treatment was started by transmitting Nux-Vom 0/3 on 3.9.73 with sufficient S.L. to be taken morning and evening,

1.10.73 :-   (1) Sugar was nil on 22.9.73 by again a trace was detected on 30.9.73.

(2) Stye on right eyelid from 22.9.73.

(3) Tingling in left sole aggr.

Transmission was put off from N.V. and Syphilinum C.M. was transmitted and S.L. given. In this way R.T. 200, Drosera

200, Gels 30, IM were transmitted according to change of symptoms and he came to Patna every month to report. His Urine Sugar was finally found nil on 10.12.73 and constitutional treatment was continued till Dec., 74 by transmitting Tuber. IM, 10M. Thuja 0/5, C.C. 0/3 C.S. 10M,Syph. C.M., R.T. 10 M and Bry 1M.

His urine and blood, sugar were examined thoroughly at Calcutta but no trace of sugar was found in Urine and blood sugar was normal.

In course of treatment, there was a return of some symptoms and his left shoulder which was stiff and painful 5 years back became stiff and painful again in April, 1974 but it could not be controlled soon and his Tingling of sole also aggravated hence he could not stick to author's treatment though he is very much satisfied with the cure of diabetes inspite of taking sweets etc. In course of treatment also, he did not follow the instructions regarding diet and used take sweets and fats etc. However he is free from the so called incurable disease the diabetes.

Case 28

Eczema

Shri Mahto aged 71 of Alamganj, Patna, who had been suffering from pertinent Eczema in his palms for 26 years, came to the author on 15.7.74 for treatment. The following troubles were noted :

(1) Eczema for 26 years.

(2) Constipation.

(3) Pain in back for 8 years.

(4) Sciatica left side for 8 years.

(5) Ring Worm.

(6) Right side hydrocele since 3 years.

Previous personal ailments :

(1) Scabies in childhood treated externally.

(2) Piles operated.

(3) Urticaria.

(4) Dog-bites thrice at 10 years age.

One of his sister died of T.B. 2 years back and another sister suffered from it 20 years back.

Mind : Miser and sympathetic.

Desires : Sweets.

Modalities :

(1)   Eczema worse in summer and wet weather. Better in winter and by warmth.

(2)   Back pain worse while sitting and rising from seat. Better by motion and warmth.

(3)   Sciatica worse on beginning of motion and better by motion and warmth.

R. Tox. was selected as similimum and it was transmitted in the 200th potency.

14.8.74   Ring-worm worse and back pain had decreased. After plussing the same remedy was transmitted.

In this way, puls. 0/10, Lyc. 0/6 and Tuber. 10M were transmitted from time to time according to symptoms. Eczema vanished by the end of 1975 but again some eruptions appeared in February, 1976 after transmitting Syph. 200 on 28.1.76 other troubles disappeared. Syph. 10M was transmitted on 24.3.76 and Eczema vanished finally by the end of July, 1976.

Case No. 29
Eczema

Master Subodh Kumar aged 17, s/o. Sri Kailash Pd. Singh of Patna, had been suffering from Eczema in purulent form on extremities for 13 years. He tried almost all pathies for longer periods without much benefit. Eruptions took the shape of deep ulcers on legs. He came to the author on 6.2.1974 and the following rubrics were collected and repertorised accordingly vide Kent's and Kishore's :

(1)   Aversion to sour things—Abies. c., Bell., Coff., Cocc., Dros., Ferr Mur., Ign., N.P., N.V., P.C., Sabad., Sul., Tuber.

(2)   Likes sweets-N.V., Sabad., Sul., and Tuber.

(3)   Abusive-N.V. and Tuber.

(4)   Itching better by Warmth-Tuber.

(5)   His grand father died of Bone T.B.

Tuberculinum was selected as similimum and it was transmitted in the 1000th potency on 6.2.74.

28.2.74 :   There was some improvement. After one plus it was again transmitted.

13.3.74 :   (1) Better in all respects.

(2) Bleeding after scratching.

Transmission from Tuber. IM was stopped and Psor. IM was transmitted as usual.

21.3.74 :   (1) Swelling on right foot from 15.3.74.

(2) Profuse bleeding after scratching.

(3) Eruptions spread to the left thigh.

(4) Itching better by warmth. Hair was detached from Psorin. and Ars. Alb. 0/6 was transmitted.

4.4.74 :   (1) Better conditions.

(2) Slight bleeding after scratching. One plus in the previous transmitting set.

20.4.74 :   Good condition. One plus more.

2.5.74 :   Very good condition. Itching much decreased. One Plus.

21.5.74 :   Slight Itching. Cavity of ulcer almost filled and healed up. One plus.

29.5.74 :   Eruptions almost disappeared.

31.7.74 :   No trouble even scars of eruptions almost vanished.

It was declared to be cured, hence transmission was made off finally. Even today (30th July, 77) he is quite well.

Case No. 30

Eczema

Dr. L.P. Singh of Patna aged 36, had been suffering from dry eczema in his feet and hydrocele in left side since long. It was reported that it was caused by Hawai Chappal. I do not know the drug for that aetiology. Hence the case was repertorised with the following rubrics :

(1)   Miser-Ars., Bry., C.C., C.F., Cina., Coloc., Lyc., Meli., M.C., Puls., Rheum. and Sepia.

(2) ↱ Better after eating-Ars., Bry., C.C., M.C., Puls. and Sepia.

(3)   Abusive-Sep.

Sep. 200 was transmitted on 8.2.70. On 17.2.70 it was reported that he was feeling vacant in his mind, thorax and abdomen. Hence it was detached the same day. S.L. was continued. On 25.2.70 it was reported that his hydrocele was soft but he was feeling tingling sensation in his feet while sitting. There was improvement in eczema. On 3.3.70 it was reported, "(1) Feeling pain in left side of his abdomen. (an old symptom), (2) Headache for the last four days and (3) 50% reduction in hydrocele". S.L. was continued. On 21.3.70 it was reported that hydrocele became normal and eczema also disappeared leaving blackish scars but there was burning sensation in urine (an old symptom).

S.L. was continued. N.V. 10 M was transmitted on 19.4.70 when he complained of some bowel trouble. It was detached on 1.5.70 when the trouble vanished. On 13.5.70 Sepia 10 M was transmitted. On 25.5.70 it was seen that the blackish scar of eczema also disappeared and he was advised to detach the hair from the medicine if there be any acute trouble.

Case No. 31
Epilepsy

Master A. Kumar, aged 15, of Gaya had been suffering from Epilepsy for three years and he had 4 attacks since March, 1970. He was brought to the author on 15.6.1970 for treatment. The case was repertorised on the following rubrics :

(1)   Aversion to sweets-Ars. alb., B.C., Causticum, Graph., Hipp., Lac. Can., M.S. N.A., Phos., Sin-n., Sulph. and Zinc.

(2)   Aversion to milk-Ars. alb., B.C., Graph., M.S., N.A., Phos., Sulph. and Zinc.

(3)   Likes Salty things-N.A., Phos. and Sulph.

(4)   Aversion to fish-Phos. and Sulph.

(5)   Cursing-Phos.

Phos. was selected as a similimum and 0/6th potency was transmitted and S.L. was given on 15.6.1970.

20.7.70 :   (1) No epileptic attack from 15.6.70 itself   but suffered from vertigo on 10.7.70.

(2) Swelling of Gums left side first then right side.

Phos. 0/6 after one plus was transmitted after detaching from the previous phial.

1.9.70 :   (1) No Epileptic attack.

         (2) Fever.

         (3) Dim vision.

         (4) Dry Eczema which had been suppressed a year earlier re-appeared.

Phos. Transmission was put off and S.L was transmitted.

21.12.70 : (1) No troubles.

         (2) Slight Eczema, Sulph. 0/20 was transmitted and S.L. was given be taken every alternate day.

5.1.71 :   No trouble, hence transmitting put off and there was no need of further treatment.

Master A. Kumar is free from trouble till today. (July, 1977).

Case No. 32
EYE TROUBLE

Shri Satya Narayan Mandal, aged 22, came to consult for his eye troubles on 14.5.1967. His eyes were watery and had sand sensation in his eyes and itching in lids which were aggravated by closing them, but constitutionally he was not a Calcarea patient. Cal, Carb 200 in globule was transmitted. He had severe aggravation. He could not move his hands even to request for disconnecting the hair. He became speechless. Then at once it was discontinued and after 5 minutes he replied in feeble voice. Then gradually he was free from his troubles.

Case No. 33
EYE TROUBLE

Smt. R. D. Devi, aged 25 years W/o Shri R. L. Nishad, Electrical Engineer of Jharia, had burning pain in her eyes with profuse lachrymation.

Puls 200. One globule was transmitted through the hair and her troubles vanished like magic.

Case No. 34
FILARIASIS

Mr. Gopal Choudhary aged 25 of Sultanganj, Bhagalpur had been suffering from Filariasis for 6 months in his left and right scrotum. On 14.4.1967 he came to consult the author for his intense bursting pain in his scrotum. He could not move without supporting his scrotum with his hand as his pain was extremely aggravated by hanging. I could not go in detail for further symptoms. On only one tip-bursting pain when hanging Vipera C. M. was tried by transmission at a distance of 10 feet. his pain vanished in no time. As soon as the remedy was brought in contact with his hair he was instantaneously free from pain.

Case No. 35
GALL BLADDER STONE

Smt. Kalawati Devi aged 42 of Champaran had been suffering from Gall-Stone. Plain X-ray was taken on 26.8.70 and it was positive. She was advised a surgical operation but she was afraid and therefore she came to author for treatment on 30.8.70 when the following salient features were noted :

1. Pain in right Hypocondrium since 1½ month, which was ameliorated by lying on right side, also by pressure.

2. Pain in the appendix region, which was ameliorated by warmth.

3. Pain in shoulder, which was ameliorated by lying on back and left side and also by pressure.

4. Sympathetic by nature.

5. Aversion to Milk.

    The treatment was started by transmitting phosphorus 0/6 on 30.8.70.

    On 14.9.70 she reported that pain of right hypocondrium was relieved but her earlier complaints coryza, loose stools had started with violent aggravation from 7.9.70. The patient was very anxious to get relief.

    Hence the transmission was put off and resumed again after a week's interval.

    Phos 0/20 and 0/25 transmitted from time to time and by end of June, 71 she got rid of stone.

Case No. 36
HEADACHE

Dr. N.K.P. Sinha, a devotee to Homoeopathic science, was reluctant to believe in transmission though he has sincere regard for the author. Once he had severe attack of headache before treating a case. On the same day, Silicea 200 was transmitted and he got immediate relief. Then the author asked him to transmit Aconite to that case (Sweety). But he touched Aconite 30 with his finger during transmitting it to Sweety, with the result he was attacked by blind headache and he fell down on the cot. Immediately he thought it to be reaction of Aconite hence he transmitted Nux Vomica 200 which gave him relief like magic.

Then Dr. Sinha was very much convinced with transmission and became a sincere devotee to it.

Case No. 37
HERNIA

Dated 22.11.68. Munmun S/o. U.K. Pathak, Pathkouli, P.S. Bagha II, Champaran, was born on 11.10.68 with congenital hernia in right side, along with diarrhoea and vomiting since birth. N.V. 2 C was transmitted. There was slight improvement in diarrhoea. On 9.12.68 Thyroidin 2C was transmitted which gave relief for 3 days only. But it did not touch hernia. On 6.1.69 Aur. Met-2C was transmitted and diarrhoea stopped by 8.1.69 with hard constipation, hence the hair was detached from the medicine. Hernia was completely normal, but constipation persisted. The stool was first hard then loose and the left side hydrocele was involved. On 3.2.69 C.C. 0/20 was transmitted but it was detached on 7.3.69 due to cough. Then there was improvement in stool but hydrocele persisted. He was crying before passing urine hence on 16.5.69 Lyco. 0/6 was transmitted and the boy was free from hydrocele and bowel troubles after detaching hair from Lyco.

Case No. 38
HERNIA

Master Rajan aged 9, son of Sri M.L. Chaudhary of Garhara, Monghyr, had been suffering from inguinal Hernia in left side from the age of 5. He was advised to get it operated, but his parents did not dare do so. He was brought to the author for treatment on 9.3.1971. The following symptoms were considered for treatment.

(1)   Likes-Milk, sweets and fat.

(2)   Dislikes-Meet, fish and sour.

(3)   Hernia left side aggravated in day and motion and ascended by the morning after rest.

There was paucity of symptoms no doubt, but treatment was started on the above rubrics by transmitting Nux. Vom. 30 and improvement started. In course of treatment there was a return to symptoms like fever opthalmia, Scabies, boils, Eczematous eruptions etc. By transmitting N.V. 200, IM & Sulphur 200, R.T. 200 and sulphur 0/6 from time to time according to change of symptoms, he was perfectly cured by the end of may 74 in about two years. He is quite well and had no relapse of hernia uptill now (July 77).

Case No. 39

HYSTERIA

A girl aged 17 of Patna had been suffering from mental trouble (hysteric fit daily between 5 and 6 p.m.) Ignatia IM was transmitted through her hair from a distance of 5 miles on the 2nd June, 1970 and she got rid of her trouble within 3 days. She is O.K. uptill now.

Case No. 40

IMPOTENCY

On 13.5.67 Mr. A. Prasad aged 35, an officer, Bhagalpur came to author for the following troubles.

(1)   Sexual weakness for 6 months.

(2)   Bowel disordered.

Previous Personal ailments, suffered from

(1) Pyorrhoea, (2) Itches and ring worm (3) Wart

(4) Malaria (5) Early onanism.

Family history : Mother suffering from Uterine cancer.

Mind :   Very miser, fault finding, malicious and liking for loneliness and memory weak.

Head :   Dandruff.

Eyes :   Normal.

Ears :   Do.

Nose :   Do.

Mouth :   Salty taste with normal thirst.

Likes :   Nothing special except warm food.

Stomach :   Flatulence aggravated from 4 P.M. A little food
              satisfied him.

Stool :   Constipation. Stool hard and long.

Urine :   Burning sometimes during urination.

M.Sex organ : Less desire. Incomplete erection.

Exts :   Palms and soles sweaty.

Sleep :   Sound, dream of flying.

Better :   Winter, motion and warm food.

Worse :   Summer and warm room.

Repertorising by : Kent.

(1)   Miser (Avarice) - Ars. Alb., Bry., C.C., C.F., Cina., Coloc.,
      Lyc., Meli., N.C., Puls., Rheum and Sepia (Page-9)

(2)   Fault finding :- Ars. Alb., C.C., Lyc., and Sep.(Page-10)

(3)   Malicious :- Ars. Alb., C.C., and Lyc. (Page-63)

(4)   Liking loneliness:- C.C. and Lyc.(page-12 Company)

(5)   Incomplete Erections :- C.C. and Lyc. (Page-695)

(6)   Dream of flying:- Lyc. (Page-1240)

      Lyco. was selected.

      Lyc. 1M.:-One globule no. 10 was transmitted. The effect
was felt on the forehead. Tingling sensation with heat on
forehead. One minute after Lyc. 200 one globule was used, he
felt hot sensation in his **chest**.

      Next time after one minute Lyc. 6 was transmitted and
sweat from his palms vanished.

      From the above effects it was concluded that Lyc. 1M. had
right direction of action hence it was given orally. On 1.6.67 it
was reported that he was 75% better. S.L. was given and after
a fortnight he was quite free from his all troubles.

      The right potency was selected by trial method here.

Case No. 41
Injury

The same day at Patna Mrs. X of Yarpur came to the dispensary of Dr. Bishwanath Prasad for treatment. Author was sitting in his chamber. People along with Dr. Bishwanath Prasad and Dr. D.N. Pathak (Homoeopaths) were curious to see the result of transmission. In short symptoms ran as follows :-

She had injury in her forehead just near her right eye with profuse bleeding. She could not move her head as her neck was stiff and was unable to open eyes due to extreme pain in her head (occiput). Led. 30 was transmitted without any effect. Then Hyper., 30 one globule no. 10 was brought in contact with that very hair. Her pain vanished like magic and she opened her eyes and moved her head freely. The spectators were surprised to see the miraculous result.

Case No. 42
Insanity

A young girl of Bombay had been suffering from mental trouble. Dr. Badh Raj of Bombay sent her hair to the author at Bettiah. Nux vom. 50 M was transmitted on the 29th May 1969 and vide his letter dated the 8th July 1969, Dr. Raj reported that she was having some relief but laziness persisted. She slept for 14 hours in 24 hours. The author detached the hair on the 15th July 1969 and informed the doctor. A report about here condition was received vide his letter dated the 4th August 1969 that she was just normal but lazy in doing domestic work. The doctor was silent for about a year. Unexpectedly the author received his letter dated the 30th July 1970 on the 8th August 1970 that the mental patient had been O.K. since a year. She had no trouble.

Case No. 43.
Insanity

The wife of Shri Singh aged 22 of Kondi Village, Patna District, had been suffering from insanity. She was brought to the author on the 2nd February 1974 for treatment. Nux vom. 0/12 was transmitted through her uprooted hair. Just after transmission, she became calm and had an attack of shivering which remained for 30 minutes. She was kept at Patna for some days to see the effect. On the 4th February 1974, she was brought again to the author. She behaved like a normal lady. She was quite well till 10th February 1974,. She was taken to Baidyanath Dham (religious place for worship) for a change, but she had a little set back and suffered from loss of sleep on the 11th February, 1974. On hearing this, plussing was done (all medicated water of the phial was thrown away and fresh distilled was added and 10 strokes were given) on the 13th February 1974. Effect was immediate. Since then she is quite normal (Kondi is about 60 Km. from Patna.

Case No. 44.
JAUNDICE

Master Supavitra Gorain aged 14, son of Sri Shankar Gorain of Govindpur, Dhanbad was seized by jaundice a week back and he was brought to the author for treatment on 2.5.77.

He had an attack of jaundice in May 76 also and he was treated by an Allopath.

The following points were noted when he was examined by the author :-

1. Jaundice.
2. White coated tongue.
3. Loss of appetite.
4. Blackish stool.
5. Enlargement of liver.
6. Weeping while narrating his symptoms.
7. Craving for sweets and salty things.

Nothing was found worth mentioning in his past personal and family history.

The case was repretorised on the following rubrics :-

1. Weeping while narrating symptoms-K.C., Medo., Puls. and Sepia.
2. Craving for sweets- K.C., Medo. and Sep.
3. Craving for Salty things-Medo.

Medo was selected as a similimum and it was transmitted in the 1000th potency. He was perfectly cured by the 3rd July 77 and the transmitting set was put off.

Case No. 45
KIDNEY STONE

Shri Shrivastava aged 5-0 Years, an Officer of Bihar Government, came to the author for treatment of Renal trouble on the 12th July 1972. Phos. 0/3 was transmitted. The author was reluctant to transmit Phos. because he had craving for sweets which contradicts it (Phos). However, the transmission was put off due to aggravation in urine. On the 17th September 1972, after reconsidering, Lyco. 0/3 was transmitted. The patient reported that he passed one stone with urine in the morning of the 7th November 1972 and he handed over it to the author. Since then he had no attack of Renal trouble. The stone looks like a plumb seed in size and shape.

Case No. 46
KIDNEY STONE

Sri B.P. Sharma aged 45, Aurangabad had been suffering from renal trouble from 1972 due to stone in the left kidney. The stone was located in the left ureter near its opening in the bladder.

He came to the author for treatment on 18.8.76 and the following salient features were noted :-

(1) Dull pain in left side with a sense of swelling which was ameliorated by lying on back and warmth; and aggravated by lying on left side and before stools.

(2) Pain in left knee from 1975 which was aggravated on ascending and rising from seat and ameliorated by warmth.

(3) Chronic dysentery from 1972 with constipation.

(4) Headache since long which aggravated with constipation

The treatment was started with the transmission of sulphur 200 on 18.8.76. On 8.10.76 he reported of violent aggravation. The old troubles-cold, cough, and breathing had reappeared from 3.9.76 along with loose stools.

The patient was very anxious to get relief at the earliest; the transmission was therefore put off and Nux. v. 200 was transmitted on 20.11.76. He was better in all respects hence five pluses were made with 10 strokes each time. He was advised to get X-ray again to find out as he seemed to have no complaint of the kidney.

On the Ist March, 1977 it was reported after a plain X-ray that no stone was detected. Hence pyelographic X-ray was taken which also failed to indicate any stone.

Itching in the whole body started and headache persisted hence transmission was made off on 1.3.77 and sepia 200 was transmitted.

He had loose stools on 11.3.77 and headache too persisted, Lycopodium 200 was transmitted on 3.4.77 after detaching 24.4.77 :-

(1)   He is free from headache since 4.4.77

(2)   He had asthmatic attacks again for a week.

(3)   He is quite free from the renal trouble.

The transmission was put off.

Case No. 47
LEUKOPLAKIA

Smt. M. Devi aged 45, wife of a Homoeopath in the interior of Darbhanga had been suffering from leukoplakia on the middle of her tongue since 1961. She underwent the modern treatment, and ultimately electric shocks were given and she got relief for some months. Again the disease raised its head after 5 months and she was advised to undergo operation which she did not dare. She was brought to the author on 8.7.73 for treatment.

(1)   Ulcer on tongue was troublesome. It was diagnosed as leukoplakia.

(2)   She had leucorrhoea since 1971.

(3)   Vertigo.

(4)   She was very weak.

Previous Ailments :

(1)   T.B. in 1954

(2)   Oedema whole body during 5th pregnancy.

(3)   Tube ligation.

(4)   Metrorrhagia eight years back.

(5)   Hysterectomy.

(6)   Malaria and quinine.

(7)   Skin disease

Mostly treated by Allopaths.

Father died of Asthma 5 years back.

Husband had been a victim to Gono. and Syph.

Mind - Orderly and fastidious.

Likes-Milk

Ars. Alb. 0/6 was transmitted on 8.7.73 and improvement started.

Every month plussing was done till oct. 73.

The whole tongue became aphathous and painful in sept. 73. In Oct. 73 the original patches on the tongue were covered with pimples.

There was difficulty in swallowing food. The throat was painful. Transmission was put off and Sycosyph. 10M. was transmitted on 18.12.73 The whole vagina became aphathous and painful. Hair was detached from the previous transmitting Set and Con 0/6 was transmitted. Plussing was done from time to time. She was free from her troubles by the end of Dec., 74.

Case No. 48
NEURALGIA

Dated 11.2.68 : Indu Bhusan Mishra, aged 32, a Sectional Officer, Gandak Project, Ram Nagar, had severe attack of neuralgic pain in left side of his face. The pain was radiating form upper left side teeth to the left ear where it was localised. The earache was highly aggravated by cold air but ameliorated by pressure and warmth. He liked high pillow and had dandruff in his head. He was miser and fastidious by nature. Ars. 200 was transmitted and he got immediate relief without return of symptom in future.

Case No. 50
PEPTIC ULCER

Sri. J.N. Pd. aged 42 of Khutouna Bazar, Madhubani had been suffering from peptic ulcer for 10 years. His weight was reduced from 90 kg. to 58 kg. inspite of all types of treatment since inception of the disease. He lost all hopes of survival and he came to the author for a trial on 12.10.1971 and the following points were noted:-

A.   (1)   Indigestion and gastric troubles with pain in stomach and heart burning

      (2)   Desire for sweets.

      (3)   Miser and desire for loneliness.

      (4)   Acid and Milk aggr.

      (5)   Appetite very less.

      (6)   Sex. desire increased.

B.   Previous personal history :-

      (1)   Obesity

      (2)   Malaria and over use of Quinine.

      (3)   Skin diseases suppressed by external applications in childhood.

      (4)   Onanism

      (5)   Warts.

C.   Family History :-

Mother and 5 other blood relations had asthma. One maternal uncle and one of his brothers were victim of epilepsy. Grand father was diabetic. One Maternal uncle died of T.B.

The case was repertorised on the following rubrics:-

(1)   Miser- Ars. alb., Bry., C.C., C.F., Cina, Coloc., Lyc., Meli., N.C., puls., Rheum, and sepia.

(2)   Likes sweets-Ars. alb., Bry., C.C., Lyc., N.C. and sep.

(3)   Sour thing aggr.- Ars., alb., N.C. and Sep.

(4)   Likes loneliness - N.C. and Sep.

(5)   Despair of recovery - Sep.

Sepia was selected as a similimum but treatment was started by transmitting Nux. Vom. 200 with a good result. In course of treatment according to symptoms N.V. 200, IM, Sepia 200, 0/6, 0/20, Sul 0/3, Cal. carb 0/3, Lyc 0/3, PULS 0/6 were transmitted from time to time and he was cured by the 22nd April 1973. His weight increased from 58 kg. to 75 kg. on 22.4.73.

He is free form his obstinate trouble and he has not taken

a single medicine orally for any trouble. He is leading a normal life.

Case No. 51
PILES

Prof. R.C. Sinha, M. J.K. college Bettiah had been suffering from blind piles since long. He had intense pain. Dr. N.K. P. Sinha transmitted Nat. Mur. 30 and Prof. Sinha was free from his trouble.

Case No 52
RHEUMATISM

The authors daughter aged 11 felt agonising cramps in her right leg when she was in bed. She was striking her leg against the bed. Author asked her to bring one globule of Rhus Tox 200 in her hand from the medicine chest. She did so. She came to bed with relief in her right leg but pain shifted to her left leg. Author ordered her to throw the globule immediately. She did so and she was free from her cramping pain and she enjoyed sound sleep in the night. Here the medicine was transmitted directly through her sensory nerve.

Case No. 53
RHEUMATISM

The author's son, Mridul Kumar aged 16, had Rheumatic trouble in his left ankle. He was feeling pain in his left knee along with headache. He is tall, lean and thin The author very much alarmed at the shifting pain from his ankle to his knee with headache, Abrotanum 200 one globule was transmitted through his hair from the chamber to him sitting in the kitchen at a distance of about 20 feet. As soon as his hair was brought in contact with the tiny globule, his headache instantaneously vanished and he felt better.

After sometimes he came to the chamber from where transmission was being done and he felt much better in the chamber. Next day he was free from all troubles and T.S was set off.

Case No. 54
SCIATICA

Shri Ambika Prasad Singh, Advocate, Bhikanpur, Bhagalpur, father of Shri N.K.P. Sinha, Munsif, Bettiah (Champaran) was suffering from sciatic pain for two and a half months, He was treated by all the eminent physicians of Bhagalpur without any relief. Ultimately the author was consulted on 14.12.68. And N.V. 200 was transmitted with immediate relief. He could move without support. On 27.12.1968 N.V. I M was transmitted which enabled him to walk down about a furlong. But it could not relieve him completely. Further symptoms came on upper surface which obliged the author to transmit K.C. 2C on 22.1.1969 which gave him complete relief and since then he has assumed his normal duty. It may be added here that he had already suffered from heart attack in the year 1958 and since then he was not in a position to lie down on left side. But after transmission of K.C. he got rid of this complaint also.

Case No. 55
SCIATICA

Sri Mundrika Singh aged 45 Nalanda district consulted the author on 20.7.74 for the following troubles :-

1. Sciatic pain on left side for the last 25 years. It started from the lumber region and extended to his left knee.

2. Filaria in his left arm since long.

3. Seminal discharge on straining at stool.

He had the history of suppression of skin diseases and injury. His father had suffered from eczema and diabetes and mother from asthma. One of his sons had T.B. glands in the cervical region.

Mind - He was abusive and weeping after anger, miser and sympathetic.

Desires - Sweets, milk and warm food.

Male sexual organ - Desire increased, pain aggravated on coition.

He used high pillow during sleep and experienced fearful dreams.

His pain was aggravated by cold, coition and beginning of

motion but ameliorated by lying on painful side, pressure and warmth.

He had been over drugged hence on 20.7.74 N.V. 0/3 was transmitted and his pain subsided. He had come to the author on a rickshaw because he was unable to move. Next morning he could walk without any help. But on 22.7.74 pain aggravated hence T.S. was put off and R.T. 0/5 was transmitted. R.T. 0/10, 0/15,Bry 0/6, Lyc 0/6, 0/12 and puls. 200 were transmitted from time to time according to symptoms and ultimately he was cured by the end of July 1975.

Case No. 56
SCIATICA

Sri Dal Bir Singh aged 38 of Patna Treasury had been suffering from Sciatica in the right side since about a month. The modern treatment could not help much; rather tingling in left foot started since 5 days, hence he came to the author on 22.3.77 for treatment. He had the following Symptoms :-

(1)   Sciatic pain aggravated in the beginning of motion and relieved by motion and warmth.

(2)   Tingling of left foot-aggravated while sitting.

(3)   He had aversion to fat.

The case was repertorised vide Kent's repertory in the following way :-

(1)   Sciatica-pain in right side-Carb. S., Cheli., Ch.S., Coloc., Dios., Lach., Lyc., Phyt., Plan., Sepia and Tell.

(2)   Better by motion Lyc.and Sepia.

(3)   Tingling aggravated by sitting. - Lyc.

22.3.77 -   Lyc. 200 was transmitted

29.3.77 -   Pain in right calf aggravated from the night of 28.3.77

             After one plus, it was retransmitted.

2.4.77 -   No improvement, hence transmission of Lyc. 200 was put off. and R.T. 200 was transmitted; pain vanished at once.

10.4.77 -   Slight pain reappeared hence hair was detached from R.T. 200 and pain again vanished like magic. After two plusses it was transmitted again.

21.4.77 - He was completely free from pain by the end of April, 1977 without any return till to-day, hence transmission was put off finally. He is quite well.

Case No. 57
SPONDYLITIS

Sri R. N. Pd. aged 40 years of Ram Nagar Diara, Patna had been suffering from spondylitis for 11 years. The modern treatment could not help him much. He came to the author on 8.8.76 for treatment and the following symptoms were noted :-

(1) The trouble started after the exposure to rain.

(2) Pain aggravated at night and after bath.

(3) Better by lying on back, motion, pressure and warmth.

(4) Likes cold milk.

(5) Greasy face.

(6) He was very weak and his weight was reduced to 45.5 kg. only.

(7) He was better in summer and worse in rainy season and winter.

He had suffered from skin diseases, liver troubles and warts. His father suffered from Jaundice and migraine and ultimately died of gout in 1942.

The totality of symptoms went in favour of Rhus Tox, to be taken morning and evening for a month.

Improvement started from the same month and weight went on increasing. R.T. 1M and 10M cured him by July, 1977 with an increase of weight by 12.5 kg.

Case No. 58
STERILITY

Smt. T.Devi aged 22, wife of Sri S.Upadhya was brought on the 7 May 1969 for treatment of sterility and various ailments. She was married on the 17th April 1962 but had no issue. After evaluation of symptoms Phos. 0/6, 0/20 and Nat. Mur. 0/20 were transmitted on different dates. M.C. did not appear after the 4th August 1969. She gave birth to a healthy female child of 10 Ibs. on the 28th April 1970.

Paralysis - The mother of Shri Singh, Patna, Bihar aged 65 years was paralysed at 4 a.m. of the 12th September 1970. She was brought in his lap by Shri Singh to the author for treatment on the 6th October 1970. Con. 200 was transmitted. In a minute she began to move her right hand and in a month she completely recovered.

Case No. 59
STERILITY

Smt. Sunayana Devi aged 22, wife of Dr. D.Pd. of Champaran district came to the author on 15.6.69 for her treatment. She had no issue though she led a married life for more than 5 years. She had been under the treatment of the modern school of medicine. The Seminal fluid of her husband was examined and found to be quite normal. She had the following symptoms -

1.   Dysmenorrhoea for 7 years.

      Pain in abdomen and lumber region aggravated during M.C., Blood was blackish, Clotted and scanty.

2.   Pain in left side of her chest since a Couple of years. It was aggr. on Coughings inspiration and lying on painful side; but ameliorated by lying on right side or back and warmth.

3.   Hard constipation since long she used to pass stool sometimes after a gap of two days. She had to sit in the latrine for a long time. Ineffectual urge was there.

4.   Vertigo on rising from seat.

      Previous Complaints :- Had Pneumonia in childhood. Injury to back by fall, measles and malaria with over uses of quinine, took vaccination regularly.

      Family history :- Her mother suffered from Rheumatism and one of her three sisters had suffered from T.B.

      Mind :- Throws things in anger, likes company, fear from darkness, obstinate. consolation, weeping on hearing music.

      Head :- Dandruff and Falling of hair.

      Mouth :- Thirstless, Dry mouth, Aphthae, Bitter taste.

      Teeth :- Caries with pain.

      Throat :- Plug like sensation and pricking pain.

      Appetite :- Normal but easy Satisfied.

      Desire :- Sweets and salty.

Aversion :- Milk and Bread

Dreams :- Snake, Child and eating.

Generalities : Better before eating and loose-clothing.

Worse : Winter and Carriage.

The remedy was selected on the following points.

1. Weeping from music - Dig., Graph., Kreos., K.M., N.C., N.S., N.V. Thuja.

2. Aversion Milk - N.C; N.S; N.V.

3. Obstinate - N.V.

N.V. 200 was transmitted on 15.6.69. She at once felt heat on her head and chest.

Sufficient Sac. L. was given for taking morning and evening.

1.7.69 - Pain in left side of her chest hence T.S.. was put off.

After this Sul 1M, Thuja M., R.T. 200, Calc carb 200, Sep 200 were transmitted from time to time according to symptoms and she conceived after the last M.C. on 18.8.70, but unfortunately she aborted on 20.10.70, in spite of her admission and care in the Motihari Hospital. However, she again came to the author on 5.12.70 and the case was again repertorised on the following rubrics.

1. Aversion to Milk - Aeth., A.C., A.T., Arn., Bell., Bry., Calad., C.C., C.S., Carls., C.V., Cina., F.P., Ign., Lac-D;, Mag-C., N.C., M.P., N.S., N.V., Phos., Puls., Rheum., Sep., Sil., Stan., Sul.,

2. Carriage <- Arn., Bry., C.C., C.V., Ign., Phos., Puls., Sep., Sil.,Sul.,

3. Obstinate - Arn., Bry., C.C., C.V., Ign., Phos., Puls., Sep., Sil., Sul.,

4. Better before eating- Bry., C.C., C.V., Ign., Phos., S 1-Sul.,

5. Sterility- C.C., Phos., Sil., Sul.,

6. Dandruff - C.C., Phos., Sul.,

7. Fear of ghost-Phos.Sul.

8. Desires Sweets - Sul.,

Hence Sul-0/20 was transmitted on 5.12.70 and C.C. 0/30 on 15.5.71 which resulted in birth of a son 12.5.72. After wards she had a daughter also on 27.10.73.

170

Homoeo Drug Energy

Case No. 60
STERILITY

W/o Sri S. Upadhaya aged 22, was brought to the author on 7.5.69 for treatment of sterility and various accompanying troubles like dysmenorrhoea, headache, colic and pain in whole body. She was married on 17.4.1962. Phos. was selected after repertorising the case and Phos 0/6 two pills were diluted into one dram phial. One hair from her head was inserted into the phial and was well corked. The phial was handed over to her with instructions to detach the hair from the phial in case of aggravation in her trouble The hair was detached on 8.5.69 due to aggravation in her colic and S.L. was continued till 14.6.69. On 15.6.69 Phos 0/20 was transmitted in the above manner which was detached on 17.6.69 due to aggravation in headache. M.C. was delayed. Nat. Mur 0/6 was transmitted on 1.7.69 and on 17.7.69 M.C. started hence the transmission was set off. The colour of blood was blackish and clotted. S.L. was continued till 23.8.69 . The next M.C. on 4.8.69 was clear. Her trouble increased hence Ign. 200 was transmitted on 24.8.69 and she got relief. It was detached on 1.9.69 when she had colic and S.L. was continued. On 11.1.69 N.M. 0/20 was transmitted as M.C. did not appear after 4.8.69 . The hair was detached on 20.11.69 and doubt for pregnancy arose in the mind. S.L. was continued. She was examined and pregnancy was declared. Biochemic medicines like Cal. Phos 6X and Kali Phos. 6X were prescribed to be used from time to time. She gave birth to a healthy female child on 1.6.70. By this time she has been blessed with two more issues.

Case No. 61
THROAT TROUBLE

Shri Satya Narain Roy aged 22 of village Sajangi, Bhagalpur, a railway employee came to consult the author for his throat trouble on 12.3.67. He was very much perturbed at the sight of blood in his sputum. The following symptoms were noted :-

Mind :- He was irritable and very sad. He was feeling as if wind were blowing on his face.

Nose :- He had catarrhal trouble. His nose was running and stopped up whenever he walked in cold open air.

Mouth :- Gums were painful to touch and bleed readily.

Throat :- When swallowing he felt sensation of a plug and of a splinter in his throat and stitching pain in throat extending to his ear. He hawked up mucus stained with blackish blood.

Stomach :- He had a great desire for sour things but aversion to fat food.

Stool :- Normal

Urine :- He had no force in urination. He had a sensation of a drop rolling down from urethra after urination.

Male Sex. Organ :- He had been a sycotic patient. his desire was increased. He had frequent seminal discharges without any dream.

Respiration :- His lungs were clear.

Modalities :- Worse from cold winds and better from warm drinks and wrapping head up. He was definitely a chilly patient. He had the history of frequent boils on his body. For his gonorrhoea allopathic drugs were consumed.

Hep. Sulph. 200 one globule was brought in contact with a hair from his head at the distance of 8 feet. He instantaneously felt a cold sensation in his forehead and nose. Then he was allowed to go home at a distance of 3 K.M. and the medicine was kept in contact with his hair. On 13.3.67 he reported that he felt much better but the effect could not reach his home. He also added that he could feel the effect of medicine within a radius of about 100 yards Then Hep. Sulph 1000 was transmitted which covered the distance of 3 K.M. On 15.3.67 he was free from throat troubles and no sign of blood was seen in his sputum. Since then his urinary trouble also vanished.

Case No. 62

Wart

The grandson of Sri B.Pd., Divisional accountant, Ganga Bridge, Patna aged 1 year had a pea sized wart on his forehead since birth. It was very tiny in size in the beginning. Gradually it increased to the size of a pea As a routine, Thuja 200 was transmitted through a hair from his head on 20.1.77. Gradually it began to decrease & by the end of Feb 77 it completely vanished and hence the transmission was put off.

REPORT ON DEMONSTRATION OF "TRANSMISSION OF DRUG-ENERGY" THOURGH SEPARATED HAIR OF PATIENT ON 12.4.69 ON THE OCCASION OF ANNUAL BIHAR STATE HOMOEO CONGRESS AT PATNA.

By

Dr. B. Sahni

Case No. 63

"Miss Kaushlaya Keshari a student of pre-science of Women's College, Patna, aged 15, had pain in her neck and lumber region which was aggravated by cold and ameliorated by pressure. She had aversion to fish, sweets and milk, and desire for cold food and high pillow.

Phos. 200 was transmitted and at once she felt giddiness and then relief in pain".

Case No. 64

"W/o Shri H.M. Das, agriculture department, had been suffering from various ailments-pain in throat, headache, colic and chest pain.

After diagnosis Sepia was selected and it was transmitted in 1M. Pain in chest and head vanished like magic".

Case No..65

"Smt. R.D.Devi aged 38 of Deoria (U.P.) had been suffering for the last Six months from various ailments like pain in the liver region, trouble arising from amenorrhoea, throat congestion due to outer growth, headache etc.

Sepia 200 was transmitted and headache from vertex vanished at once but it remained in other parts. Then Sepia 1 M was transmitted which aggravated her vertigo. She vomited and then got relief".

Case No. 66

"Shri G.Roy aged 70 had been suffering from serious type of asthma for the last 20 years. When he appeared before Dr. Sahni, he was panting for breath due to asthmatic attack. He was a hot patient and fan gave him some relief.

Apis 200 was transmitted and his paroxysm of asthmatic attack vanished like magic. The spectators were surprised to see the effect of transmission".

Case No. 67

"Shri D. Singh had been suffering from headache, cold and cough, and pain in chest.

Bryonia 200 was transmitted and he got relief in his trouble within a second"

Case No. 68

"Shri G. Prasad aged 36, had cold sensation on his vertex for 16 years, burning sensation in eyes for the same period, giddiness and other complaints.

Lachesis 200 was transmitted. He felt flash of heat in the body and giddiness vanished at once. He also reported the feeling of taste of spirit in his mouth".

Case No. 69

"A student of Homoeo College had seminal weakness but there was no trouble at the time of demonstration. His palms and soles were sweaty."

"Acid Phos, 200 was transmitted and he felt some giddiness and slight pain in his head".

Case No.70

"Another Student of the same Homoeo College had the same type of Seminal trouble with hard constipation. At the time of demonstration he had no trouble.

Silic. 200 was transmitted and his palms began to perspire within a minute".

The demonstration was followed by a talk on 13.4.1969 by Dr. Sahni which was really very convincing and attractive.

(Sd.)
D.C. Kern,
15.4.70
(Dr. D.C. Kern)
President,
Bihar State Homoeo Congress,
All India Institute of Homoeopathy
Member,
Homoeo Advisory Committee
(India Govt.)
Patna-3.

Report of Demonstration :-

REPORT ON DEMONSTRATION OF TRANSMISSION OF DRUG-ENERGY ON 29-3-1970 ON THE OCCASION OF THE 14TH ANNUAL SESSION OF BEHAR RAJYA MISTANBHOJAN BIKRETA SANGH BY THE

Dr. B. Sahni

"The 14th annual session of Behar Rajya Mistan-Bhojan Bikreta Sangh was held on Sunday the 29th March, 1970 at Zowatika Hall (Rotary Club) Gaya under the Presidentship of Shri Radhey Shyam Modi".

"Over one thousand delegates and participants attended the conference".

Homoeo Ratna, Dr. B. Sahni, Patna was specially invited on the occasion to give a demonstration of transmission of homeopathic medicines through the detached hair from the head of the patient. He gave the following demonstration before the large gatherings and thereafter spoke on the theory of his research. He replied to volleys of questions put forward from the public present as well as from the homoeopaths gathered there"

Case No. 71

"Shrimati Balwant Kaur (40) Mir Abu Saleh Rd.

Outsider suffering from pain in right knee for the last 3-

4 days, had also pain in back etc. Rhus.Tox. 1 M touched with her detached hair. No action. Bell. 200 used but no action. Then Rhus. Tox. 30. She began to feel weakness and sensation of trembling. The hair was detached and the patient discharged".

Case No. 72

"Shri S.N. Tripathi (36) New Godown Gaya.

Pain in rectum while passing stool. Suffering for the last 10-12 years. The pain lasts for 3-4 hours after stool and subsides after taking rest. Sometimes pain rises at night making him restless and sleepless. The detached hair from his head was touched with a globule of Tuberculinum 1 M. No action, then Sulphur 30 was used. No change. Then upon suggestion of Dr. Vishwanath Prasad Nitric Acid 200 was used. He got relief. The hair was detached and the patient was advised to take Nitric Acid 200 orally".

Case No. 73

"Shrimati Shail (20), Chand Chaura, Gaya.

Pain in loin-pain in stomach 24 hours on respiration. No appetite-Rhus. Tox. 30. No relief. Colocynth 30. No action. The patient was discharged".

Case No. 74

"Shri Tribeni Ram.

Suffering from pain in teeth. The detached hair was touched with a globule of China 200 (Prescription by Dr. Vishwanath Prasad). The patient got immediate relief and he was discharged".

Case No. 75

"Shri Prabhat Kumar, (15) Member of the Sangh:

Headache for last 2-3 days, thick yellowish discharge from nose-one nostril closed alternately. Silicea 200 was prescribed. The detached hair of the patient was touched with a globule of the medicine. The patient got relief within a minute".

Case No.76

"Shri Gulam Jillani (38).

Pain in back and knee of left side only. Gas in Stomach at 4 P.M. Urine turbid. Lyco. 30-felt relief in gas trouble only".

Case No. 77

"Shri Rameshwar Prasad Gupta, Member of the Sangh.

Feels gas in stomach-on taking food. No relief from Bryonia 30. The detached hair was touched with Nux Vom. 200. Got relief".

Case No. 78

"Shri Sita Ram.

Pain in the right leg. The detached hair of the patient touched with a globule of Rhus. Tox. 200. Got relief in few minutes".

Case No. 79

"Shri Suresh Prasad Gupta (20), Member of the Sangh.

Got contusion injury in middle finger of his right hand. Painful and inflammed. The detached hair was touched with a globule of Arnica Mont. 200. The patient got relief in a few seconds.

Case No.80

"Shri Komal Sao (55), Mangla Gauri, Member of the Sangh.

Trouble in respiration on rising in the morning. Pain in both knees, trouble below the knees (on movement), while sitting and watery discharge from eyes. The detached hair was touched with a globule of Bry. 30. Got relief. (Prescribed by Dr. Vishwanath)".

Case No. 81

"Shri D.P. Singh, Asst. Sub-Inspector, Kotwali.

Pain in abdomen-Dysentery.

The detached hair was touched with globule of Nux. Vom. 200. Got relief in a few minutes.

This note was prepared and submitted by Dr. Vishwanath Prasad, Secretary, Behar Rajya Mistan Bhojan Bikreta Sangh, Gaya branch and Secretary All India Institute of Homoeopathy (Regd.) Gaya Branch, Veez Hotel Gaya.

Sd/-
Vishwanath Prasad,
29.3.70"

EXPERIMENTS ON ANIMALS

Case No. 82
ANOREXIA

The author's cat after giving birth to 4 kittens on the 30th November, 1971 fell ill on the 10th December, 71. She was sitting in a sad mood closing her eyes in one corner of the house and did not respond to any calls. She had complete loss of appetite. The kittens were mewing continuously which disturbed our sleep in the night and the author thought of treating her next morning but failed to do so till 14.12.71. On the 15th December, 71, the author determined to the needful to relieve her suffering. There was paucity of symptoms. However, some rubrics were extracted from the situation. Milk, bread and fish were offered one by one but she could not touch them, hence it was inferred that she had aversion to fish and milk though cats are fond of these two items of food. In the same way it was inferred that she was indifferent to her kittens, because she ignored their mewing for 5 days. The case was repertorised vide Kent's Repertory in the following way :

1. Aversion to fish-Colch., Graph., Guar, N.M., Phos., Sulphur and Zinc.

2. Aversion too milk-Guare. Phos. and sulphur.

3. Indifferent to Children (Kitten) - Phos.

Phosphorus runs through all the rubrics hence it was selected. One tiny pill (No. 10) of phos 0/6 was dissolved into one damp phial of distilled water and transmitted through one hair from her face.

The effect was miraculous. As soon as the hair was brought in contact with that solution, she began to move as if searching a food. Milk was offered and she took it greedily. Bread was also taken with good cappetite. The same night she began to attend to her kittens' calls and since then she has been quite well.

Case No. 83
BLOODY URINE OF A HEIFER

A crossbred black heifer of 3½ years of age (Prize- winner) belonging to Dr. Ram Swaroop Sinha, joint Director Animal Husbandry, Bihar, Patna was pregnant for three months. It got complaints of bloody urine with temperature 103, loss of appetite, less frequent urination, dullness etc. The heifer was treated with Veterinary medicines, injections etc. first, but the bloody urine persisted. A hair from the tail of the said heifer was brought to the author and Apis 200 was transmitted through that hair on 4.9.77. The bloody urine got clear in 3 days time, and dullness, appetite and frequency of urination improved. Within a week, the sick heiferr got normal in all respects and Transmission was set off on 20.9.77.

Case No. 84
COLD

In May, 1967 author's cow was attacked by sever cold. She was sneezing frequently. Copious water discharge was coming out from her nose and eyes. She was restless and thirsty. She had appetite for fodder. She was better in the morning but worse in the evening. He was tempted to try "Transmission". One hair from her tail was taken out and Allium Cep. 200 one globule was brought in contact with it at a distance of 12 feet from the cow. The remedy had immediate effect. Her sneezing was aggravated and she could sneeze every second for some minutes. Then the hair was disconnected from the remedy. To his utter surprise she was free from the trouble in two hours.

Case No. 85

INJURY

On the 31st May, 76 the author was called in by one of the top officers of Bihar Govt. for consultation. While the case history was being taken down, his bitch named Shiva came into the drawing room limping on its 3 legs only and its left foreleg was dropped at its wrist. On enquiry it was learnt that it had a sprain 26 days back and was treated without relief. The author was interested to treat it with injury drugs hence one globule of Arnica 200 was transmitted as usual through her up-rooted hair. Just after half an hour, the bitch began to try to keep its affected limb on the ground but could not do so.

On the 6th June, 76 there was some improvement but limping still persisted. The hair was taken out of the Arnica solution and Ruta 30 was transmitted. Shiva got well and so its hair was taken out of solution on the 30th August, 76.

Case No. 86

MASTITIS

On the 28th May, 1973 the author had a chance to visit Sri. R. Upadhya's village, in the Naubatpur Block, Patna. Sri. Upadhya requested him to do something for his buffalo whose one of the udders was going to be lost due to mastitis after parturition. Very scanty watery milk along with yellow and granular pus was coming out. One hair from her tail was brought to Patna from Naubatpur, a distance of about 30 K.M. and on the following day Silicea 200 was transmitted as usual. Next time the author went there to attend a meeting on 16.6.73. Sri Upadhya reported that pus was not coming out any more and milk was scanty but normal in colour. Hair was detached from Silicea solution and puls. 200 was transmitted on the 19th June, 73. It had a wonderful effect. Quantity of milk began to increase and by the end of July, 73 it was quite normal hence transmission was stopped on the 14th August, 73.

Case No. 87

TUMOUR

Sri B.P. Jhunjhunwala's Alsatian dog had an orange size tumor on its neck for a fortnight which was painful. It looked fat and sad, ɔasking silently in the sun. It had no appetite. It was treated by the veterinary surgeon without much relief. There was paucity of symptoms no doubt, but examining the physical features of the dog, the author thought of transmitting Cal. carb. He asked for a hair from his body and he took it to his residence at Bettiah at a distance of about 18 K.M. from Chanpatia Next morning one tiny pill of Cal. 10M. was dissolved in one dram phial and transmitted through its hair. The tumor disappeared within a month.

CASES BY Dr. B.BN. SAKSENA, AJMER
Case No. 88

"22.1.68 : Shrimati Susila Devi aged 25, wife of Shri Kamal Jee, Clerk in Metal Works, Muhalla Chandiki, Taksal, Jaipur, had been suffering from measles for 4 days. The face was red with 103 degree temperature. Severe headache in temples, Upper portion of the body was heated like fire etc.

One hair from the head of the patient was taken by the root and placed on the table at a distance of six feet from the patient. Bell. 200 was brought in contact with the hair. The result was miraculous. Headache and fever vanished instantaneously. The other symptoms too began to decrease within four minutes. Measles began to subside. The same action was repeated next day when she was free from measles and fully cured".

Case No. 89

"24.1.1968 : Shri Merri Lal aged 18, S/o Shri Mihilal, a messenger in the Secretariat, Government of Rajasthan, Jaipur residing in Muhalla Brohampuri, Jaipur, was suffering from pain in the right side of his chest which was aggravated during breathing and coughing. The temperature was 103 degrees. He was worse from movement and better by rest. There was tendency to lie down and sleep. It was diagnosed as severe case of Pneumonia".

"Bryon. 200 in globule was transmitted by bringing the medicine in contact with his hair at a distance of 8 ft.. The pain vanished within a second and he was miraculously cured within minutes at the spot".

Case No. 90

"27.1.1968 : Shrimati Mira Devi, W/o Shri M. Behari Srivastava of Nasirabad, Dayal Ka Bara, Srinagar Road, Ajmer, had been suffering from severe colic for the last twenty five days. The case was tried by some physicians and admitted into the Civil Hospital, Ajmer, for about 15 days and then was handled by a renowned Allopathic practitioner without any benefit. She was in a precarious condition when she was brought to me. On examining her in such a condition I thought to treat the case by administering the Homoeo medicine Gels. 200 through the above method with the result that the case got a little amelioration only. Then I had to turn to my own discovered system of treatment "EFFECTS THROUGH RADIATION PRODUCED BY EXTERNAL USE OF HERBS AND PLANTS from a distance-MEDICO-PSYCHOTHERAPY. I tried Achyranthus aspera plant from a distance but she did not get much benefit. Then again I took the help of TRANSMISSION. Mag. Phos. 200 was transmitted through the hair of patient at distance of 6 ft. to utter astonishment of every one. The patient was cured within no time like magic".

Case No. 91

"30.6.68 :Shri Gopi Chand aged 20, resident of Shri Lalkis, Ajmer, was suffering from fever and congestive headache with throbbing pain. The face was red, better from pressure or tight bandage-sudden vomiting. It appeared to have been affected by the sun.

Bell. 200 was transmitted through his hair separated from his head from a distance of 10 ft.The fever and other troubles subsided and fully cured in one hour".

Case No. 92

"8.7.68 : Shrimati Shanti Devi aged 20, resident of Gujardharti Muhalla, Ajmer, had been suffering from painful retention of urine with intense burning sensation for three days. She got no relief in two days by my own Ayurvedic treatment. Canth. 200 was transmitted and the result was miraculous. She passed urine for the first time with comfort and only a little sensation, which too vanished in her next urination within two hours".

Case No. 93

"9.8.68 : A baby aged 8 months was suffering from Diarrhoea during teething. She was restless with pain specially during night. She could not keep mum even for a minute. Irritative cry before and after stool. She was carried about here and there. Cham. 30 was transmitted and she got immediate relief and enjoyed sound sleep during the night".

Case No. 94

" 26.8.1968 : Shrimati Bambia aged 26, resident of Angarpur, Ajmer, was suffering from vomiting and fever since two days. ipecac. 30 was transmitted with a little relief on 27.8.1968. Ipecac. 200 was transmitted and she got immediate relief and permanent cure".

Case No. 95

"29..8.1968 : Shri Jaikishore, aged 20, resident of Nasirabad, Ajmer, was suffering from pain in the right arm during rest. Pain was subsided when moving about and working for the last six days. Rhus. Tox. 200 in globule was transmitted through his hair at the distance of 10 ft. He got relief immediately".

CASES BY DR. K.P. SRIVASTAVA AJMER
Case No. 96

" On 26.11.68 my son, Master Govind got high fever of 104^0 with pain in his left side of the chest. I separated hair from his head and touched Bryonia 200 from a distance of ten feet and waited for the result. Within 4 or 5 minutes it was observed that the pain vanished and temperature came down to 98^0 and within one hour he came in normal condition hale and hearty. This, my first successful test trial made me firm that the energy of Homoeo medicine can be transmitted through hair and the discovery made by Dr. B. Sahni is based on some fundamental scientific lines".

Case No. 97

"Again on 2.12.68, my son suffered with 103^0 fever and other connecting symptoms to Homoeo medicine, Belladonna which was tried in 200th potency by touching his hair from a distance of 12 feet and relief was observed like magic within 2 to 3 minutes.

These two successful experiments encouraged me to try this method further. In other cases of various ailments the result was marvellous".

CASE BY DR. RAM EKBAL SINGH

Chanpatia,

16.3.1969

Respected Dr. B. Sahni,

Pranam.

Case No. 98

You will be again pleased to know the second example of the success of your method that in the night of 20.2.1969 Dr. Malti Sinha, my wife felt severe pain in her head. She was almost unconscious due to pain. I remembered the method invented by you and applied. I transmitted Glon. 6 through her uprooted hair and astonished to inform you that the next minute she was smiling. Pain disappeared. She got complete relief and she is quite okay now. From that day I am a blind follower of your method.

Yours,

(Sd.) Ram Ekbal Singh,

B.E.E.O. Chanpatia,

Regd. Homoeopath.

By. Dr. D.N. Ramachandran
M.D.E.H., Coimbatore.

Case No. 99

1.   "The very simple experiment was made by me on Friday last(5.8.77). A young girl of sixteen (my own grand daughter had colic during her menstrual period. As soon as she informed me, I got hair form her head-a pretty long one, enclosed it in a small vial with a solution of Belladonna 6X in water, and closed the top with its metal cap. The hair remained submerged in the solution. In ten minutes she got full relief. There was no antenna of the hair outside".

"What, however, I did was this. The bottle with the solution and hair was given a good shake-up for a minute and then left on my table. The patient was far away at home. In 10 minutes she was asleep on the floor fully relieved of the excruciating pain".

Case No. 100

2.   "I was forced last Friday, the 19th August 1977, by another experiment, the patient being my eldest grand-daughter. She complained of acute menstrual pains last Friday morning I sent for doses of Bell. 6 from a local Homoeopath having his clinic 10 houses away in the same street as mine, he had with him only Bell 30 in stock and sent me 2 doses of it (each having 3 globules).

Grand-daughter refused to pluck a hair of her head on sentimental grounds, it being a Friday. So, I made the solution of one dose of 3 globules in a vial (small one) and asked her to spit enough quantity of her saliva which she did".

"Lid was tightened on to mouth of the vial and kept on my table . In 20 minutes the pain gradually decreased and Completely vanished.

Note by the author :- (i) Regarding saliva it may be referred to pages 35-36 of the first edition of the book. "Homoeopathic dynamic medicine can be transmitted to a patient in any corner of the world just like radio system through the medium of *any natural belonging* to the patient. Subsequently it was experimented thoroughly on blood, sputum, saliva, photo, voice etc.

(ii) Regarding submersion of hair into solution it can be said that radiation from T.S. being electromagnetic in nature can easily penetrate the solution and the vial.

The author would like to cite some more cases of some of the followers of Drug Transmission.

By Dr. Parmeshwar Sah. B. Sc. (Bio.) D.M.S. (Hons.) Pat.

Case No. 101

Hardness of hearing due to perforation of Tympanic membrane.

Shri D.N. Choudhary, Patna came to my clinic on 25.12.74 along with his son, Shri V.K. Choudhary aged 23 years, for treatment. Shri V.K. Choudhary was suffering from impaired hearing since 1964. Besides this he suffered from enlarged tonsils also which were operated on 2.11.74 but even after operation there was no improvement in his impaired hearing. Shri D.N. Choudhary was completely frustrated about complete cure of his only son. Shri V.K. Choudhary was unable to hear the tickling sound of wrist watches as also unable to hear the telephonic call. Even if sitting side by side one has to call him loudly and then he could be able to hear and respond.

Family history-Grand father died of Diabetes. Grand mother was suffering from gout, uncle suffered from paralysis and Father's sister died of Dropsy. Out of seven sisters four have died.

On the basis of following mental and physical symptoms of the patient, Merc. sol was selected as medicine (according to Kents Repertory) :

1. Habit of Masturbation.
2. Hurry.
3. Obstinate.
4. Habit of fault findings.
5. Vindictive.
6. Desire for meat.
7. Perspiration staining yellow.
8. Stains of perspiration difficult to wash off.

9.   Humorous.

10.   Perforation of membrane Tympani.

11.   Tongue fissured.

12.   Caries of teeth.

13.   Salivation during sleep sometimes.

Since Shri V.K. Choudhary had taken a number of allopathic medicines so at first he was transmitted Nux. Vom. 200 according to Sahni method of Transmission. He was advised to report again after one month but Shri Choudhary reported on 3.1.75 and informed that on 26.12.74 an abscess was formed on his left knee, which was painful. 10 strokes given in the transmitting set and much relief was felt by the patient in the pain. He was advised not to use any medicine for the abscess. He again reported on 30.1.75 and informed that since 27.1.75 he is hearing the tick-tick sound of watch and also the sound of telephone. One plussing was done.

Again on 10.3.75 and 27.4.75 one plussing more on each date was done, Shri Choudhary reported that his left ear is now alright but he is hearing less from his right ear.

He complained of some trouble only in right ear. On 21.9.75 Nux-Vom was detached and Merc sol-200 was transmitted. Improvement in right ear was reported on 20.11.75 and one more plussing was done on 22.12.75 and 1.2.76, plussings were done one after another.

Shri Choudhary reported on 4.4.76 that he is now alright. Accordingly transmission was stopped. Shri Choudhary got himself examined by an ear specialist who also told him that his both ears were without perforation.

One point which is worth mentioning is that throughout the period of treatment no placebo was given to the patient.

Case No. 102
A CASE OF WARTS ON FACE

Shri B. Prasad of Lohia Nagar, Patna consulted me at my clinic on 17.2.76 for several warts on his face. He reported that he had already taken Thuja and some other homoeopathic drugs but the warts did not yield to them. There were altogether ten in number, all of them on his face. He used to get them removed

surgically every month. His symptoms were taken as follows :
(1) obstinate, (2) filthy habits, (3) Aversion to acids, (4) desire for
salty things. His constitutional remedy was selected as Sulphur.
Sulphur 50 M was transmitted to him through Sahnis Method.
There was no improvement till 15.3.76. The potency of the drug
was raised by a plussing. On 15.4.76 sulphur C.M. potency was
transmitted. He reported on 19.4.76 that 2 and 3 swollen glands
had appeared in both the armpits respectively which were very
painful. A few strokes given to the transmitting set relieved him
of the pain immediately. On 15.5.76 a few of the warts had fallen
down. The potency of the drug was raised by a plussing on
17.6.76 and he had no wart left on his face. The transmission
was continued till 20.7.77. Hence the patient was cured only by
transmission of homoeo drug energy. Oral administration of
drug was not essential at any stage of treatment.

Case No. 103
EPILEPSY CURED

Mr. A. Nath, 12 years was suffering from Epileptic fits
since Dec. 1973. Prior to this attack he had got injury in his head
and had suppressed itch with external application. Immediately before the attack he used to have twitching of the eyes, his
whole body trembled, his body got stiffened then he used to fall
down unconsciously and froth oozed from his mouth. He used
to have two attacks in a day and two at night usually.

His Grand father was a victim to syphilis and sycosis. One
of his uncles had tuberculosis and the other had epilepsy.

Nux Vomica was selected to be his similimum with Kent's
Repertory on the following points :

1.   Aversion to acids.
2.   Obstinate.
3.   Malicious.
4.   Fault findings.
5.   Weeping after anger and
6.   Despair of recovery.

Nux Vomica-200 was transmitted to the boy through
detached hair from his head on 26.10.74. Immediately the boy
felt a pleasant lightness in head and relief in sore throat. On
22.11.74 the boy reported to have some mild attacks since then.

The potency was raised by a plussing.

The boy visited my clinic to report once in a month and every time he had improvement. The drug potency was raised by plussing every month. He had reported that he did not have any attack since 9.12.74. On 2.4.75 he developed parotid gland which was painful. He suffered from dysentery on 13.8.75. These troubles yielded to plussing of the same remedy. The transmission of drug was discontinued on 6.10.75 when he reported that he had no trouble left, and syco-syphilinum 1000 was transmitted on 10.11.75. The treatment was closed on the request of the parents as no trouble was left now.

The boy is alright since then.

Case No. 104
A CASE OF BRAIN TUMOUR

Mr. A. Singh was suffering from left sided paralysis and Brain tumor. He did not respond to the treatment of a few reputed doctors of the modern medical therapy at Patna. He came under my treatment on 4.7.74. His troubles were (1) Hemiplegia, (2) Vertigo, (3) Diabetes, (4) Sleeplessness after midnight, (5) Blind Piles, (6) Ringworm at thigh and (7) Constipation.

His penis had been amputated in the year 1959 due to gangrene which was later diagnosed by biopsy to be cancerous. Family history was full of T.B. and cancer. Nux Vomica was selected as his constitutional remedy with the help of following rubrics. Abusive and cursing temperament, Micious, factor finding, weeping after anger and oversensitive.

Nux Vomica-200 was transmitted to him through a hair detached from his head. Immediately he felt relief in his headache and also in the pain of the back and ankle

On 15.7.74, there was marked improvement in his paralysed parts.

On 16.8.74 he was able to walk and could raise his left hand to some extent. The potency was increased by plussings.

On 22.9.74 he reported to have had sound sleep which he had lost 14 years back. There was no trace of paralysis. The potency of the drug was raised by plussing.

On 18.10.74 he could walk up to my clinic and had

regained health. Now the only trouble left was that on raising left arm he felt pain in the left shoulder.

The patient reported on 14.11.74 that a deep X-ray taken at Darbhanga Medical College Hospital had revealed that nothing was left of the brain tumor but the V.D.R.L. was still positive.

The same drug was continued for some months with occasional plussings. On 10.2.75 the aforesaid remedy was detached and syco-syphilinum was transmitted in 10 M potency for further two months. On 15.4.75 he reported about the aggravation in his Ring worm from 14.3.75. Syco-syph. C.M. was transmitted for some months followed by occasional plussings and there was no trouble left. He reported on 20.6.75 that he was alright. Accordingly transmission was stopped.

<h3 style="text-align:center">Case No. 105</h3>
<h3 style="text-align:center">A CASE OF IRIS PROLAPSUS</h3>

Sumita aged 3 years was brought to my clinic for treatment of prolapsus of iris in both her eyes on 3.12.73. She had not shown any response while in the treatment of the orthodox specialists. She was sickly and pot bellied. Her eyelids, fingers and feet were swollen. Feet were icy cold to touch. She used to keep her eyes closed which exuded yellowish mucus. She was also discharging thin white mucus from nose.

It was reported that she had a great desire for earth eating and also suffered from diarrhoea.

Her guiding symptoms were : (1) Obstinate, (2) Aversion, (3) desire for earth and salty things (4) used to lie on abdomen.

Calcarea carb was chosen to be her medicine with the help of Kent's Repertory but as she had taken huge quantity of earth and also high antibiotics, I decided to administer Nux. Vomica 200, solution of which was prepared in a vial and it was transmitted to her through a hair detached from her head. Next time it was reported that she had left taking earth. The hair was detached from Nux. Vomica. On 11.12.73. Physostigma 30 was transmitted to her on the advice of Dr. B. Sahni. As a result, a discharge from her ears reappeared on 13.12.73. On 28.12.73 she had no swelling left on her eyes. The transmitting set was given a plussing. The swelling over her feet also showed improvement on 5.1.74. On 5.2.74 it was seen that there was no discharge from her eyes and she could open her eyes in the dark. She suffered from dysentery on 24.1.74. The potency was again raised by a plussing. Her dysentery got well and now she suffered dry cough with occasional vomiting. On examination on 25.3.74 it was seen that she had regained her lost eye sight. On 24.5.74 she was reported to have some cough left and had again started to take earth. Physostigma was detached from her hair and Calcarea Carb 200 was transmitted and on 22.5.77 it was reported that she had expelled a round worm with stool and also that she had left taking earth. The treatment was continued for sometime and she got healthy.

Case No. 106
Eczema

Shri R.L. Singh aged 35 years of Naubatpur came to my clinic on 24.11.74 for treatment of Eczema. He told that he was under treatment of eminent skin specialists for a pretty long time but of no use. He was suffering from it since 1956 and the disease has covered his whole body i.e. throat, chest, armpits, face, abdomen, waist, back, elbows, wrists, palms, soles and penis as well. At some places specially at neck and chest the Eczema was reddish and itching. These places were converted into white patches and whole body was looking like that of a leucoderma patient. Besides this he was suffering from other ailments also.

Family history : Father and mother suffered from Asthma.

Two sisters—Eczema.

Third sister—Insanity.

Mother-in-law—Asthma.

Eczema aggravated by wetting, cold, excessive perspiration, and undressing, and relieved by warmth. He has taken besides allopathic medicines, Sulphur, Graphites, Natrum Mur. etc. The Eczema was dry.

On the following mental and physical symptoms of the patient Arsenic alb. was selected according to Kent's Repertory :

1.   Avarice.
2.   Fear of insanity.
3.   Obstinate.

4.   Itching aggravates after undressing.

5.   Itching-must scratch until it bleeds.

Since Shri Singh had taken a large quantity of medicines, hence at first Nux. Vom 200 was transmitted through one of his detached hair. Before transmission of medicine the patient was feeling light headache which vanished after two minutes of transmission. The patient first felt a sensation in his head which was ultimately felt in his soles. Later on there was no such sensation. One plussing each day was done on 25.12.74, 26.1.75 and 26.2.76 due to which the Eczema aggravated. So the patient was restless all through. But within ten days most of the patches of Eczema vanished and the colour of the skin was normal. The transmission of Nux. Vom. was stopped. On 4.3.75 Arsenic Alb. 200 was transmitted to the patient but it was reported on 4.4.75 that there was no improvement in Eczema. Arsenic Alb. 1 M was transmitted on 5.4.75 and one plussing was given on 11.5.75. Arsenic Alb. 10 M was then transmitted on 11.6.75. On 9.7.75 much improvement was visible in Eczema. Since then no report was received from the patient and as such transmission of medicine was stopped. However on 20.2.77 Shri Singh came to my clinic in connection with the treatment of another patient. On enquiry about his Eczema, he informed that he was completely cured. The patient is alright till now.

Case No. 107
Case by Dr. Bishwanath Prasad
ENLARGEMENT OF MAMMAE IN MALE

Enlargement of Mammary glands in girls during adolescence is a natural phenomenon which is a sign of their puberty, but sometimes enlargement of mammae in boys is also found. This is a very peculiar disease. Boys suffering from this disease feel shy in disclosing their trouble and physicians also generally do not find its accurate remedy. In my view the main cause of this disease is malfunctioning of Pituitory, the master gland.

One such case is reproduced below from my case records :

On 11.3.75 Master A.K. Verma aged 14 years, son of a local Homoeopathic practitioner was brought to me for treatment of his following troubles :

(1)   Enlargement of both mammae for last two years.

(2)   Hardness of hearing in right ear, after an attack of typhoid some 5 years back.

(3)   Constipation-no urge in morning, urge only after taking meal.

(4)   Grinding of teeth during sleep.

There was history of typhoid, dysentery and skin eruptions previously but nothing worth mentioning in family history.

In mental symptoms weeping after anger, aversion to company taciturn, hurry, obstinacy, starting from sleep were prominent. Had desire for sweets, milk and meat. Weight 35 Kg. only.

His remedy was selected on following points :

Weeping after anger-Arn., Bell., Nux V., Plat.,

Taciturn-Arn, Bell, Nux V, Plat.

Obstinate-Arn, Bell., Nux V.

Hurry-Bell., Nux V.

Desires milk-Nux V.

Hence Nux V. 0/5 was transmitted through his hair on 11.3.75.

On 12.4.75 he reported that he had no constipation, slight improvement in hearing trouble and also in enlargement of mamma. Weight 36 Kg. Hence transmitted the same remedy after one plussing.

Next time he came after three months on 16.7.75 and reported that for the last few days he had pain in eyes with lachrymation, which < by reading. On examination there was no > in mamma enlargement. The weight was also constant i.e. 36 Kg. only.

Hence transmission of Nux V. was stopped and pituitrin. 200 was transmitted.

The patient turned up next time on 14.9.75 and reported that the troubles had gone. He had fever twice last month. There was marked > in enlargement of mamma. Weight 37.5 Kg. Hence the same remedy was transmitted after plussing.

On 16.10.75 he reported cough and cold since 14.10.75. The mammary glands were hardly perceptible. Weight 38.5 Kg. Hence retransmitted the same remedy after one more plussing.

This time the patient did not turn up for months together. His father informed on 6.7.76 that he was luckily free from the trouble. On 24.7.76 when the patient appeared for examination it was found that there was actually no trace of the mammary glands. Weight was 41.5 Kg. Hence detached transmission of Pituitrin.

Dr. A.C. Jha, M.Sc. Ph.D.
Department of Chemistry.
B. N. College, Patna and Homoeopath.

In order to test the reliability of Sahni's method of transmission of homoeo drug from a distance, I followed his method in the treatment of a number of patients suffering from various troubles. Only a few cases are given below from my case records. In every case aqueous solution of selected remedy (prepared by dissolving 1-2 globules in 1 dram of water kept in a phial) and patient's hair have been used for transmission and 5-10 strokes have been given to the phial in order to initiate the reaction. Effect of transmission (E.T.) is given under individual case.

Case No. 108
COLD AND COUGH

A child (my sister's grand son) aged about 2 was a chronic patient of cold and cough. Allopathic treatment could suppress his trouble for short period but again it relapsed. The child along with my sister came to my village to attend a marriage function where I was also present. I have to come to Patna and the patient had to go home after five days. Thinking about possible aggravation in trouble of the patient in absence of a Doctor after oral administration of selected drug, I followed Dr. Sahni's transmission process in which aggravation could be easily checked by detachment of hair from the drug. Hepar Sulphur 200 was transmitted on the basis of following symptoms on 18.4.76 :

1.   Frequent thin stool with smell.

2.   (a) Repeated attack of cold and cough;

         (b) Respiration difficult, stertorous.

3.   < latter part of night and morning.

4.   Chronic skin eruption-boil on the lower part of the body which easily suppurates.

(E.T.) EFFECT OF TRANSMISSION

1.   A rise in temperature of body observed within 1 minute after transmission.

2.   All the troubles < on 23.4.76 hence hair was detached according to direction.

3.   > On 25.4.76

4.   On 21.4.76 the boy was reported to be free from all the troubles.

Case No. 109
ABSCESS

Shri Bhola Sahu, Demonstrator in Chemistry, B.N. College, Patna aged about 40 was suffering from an abscess which was so painful that he passed two sleepless nights and hence he came to me to have some medicines so that his trouble be immediately ameliorated. He was suffering from fever also. Heper Sulphur 200 was transmitted in another room, where he was not present :

(1)   Oversensitiveness in the painful part and

(2)   < Evening and night were the indications to select the remedy.

E.T. (1)   Change in temperature of the head was observed.

(2)   Reported definite > within seven minutes on the spot.

(3)   After 20 minutes he sat properly on the chair, pressing the abscess and even ready to burst it. I intervened, 'Bhola babu, 20 mts. earlier, you have not allowed me to touch the abscess now how do you dare to burst it?". He simply laughed, walked in the room, felt easy and accepted that really there was no need to take medicine. He left my residence and went to his house which is about 4 K.M. away from my house. But transmission was already going on in my room.

(4)   The same day the absess itself bursted at 11 P.M. and patient had a sound sleep. But transmission was still continued.

(5)   After three days he reported another abscess and pain in hands and legs (an old trouble). So transmission was stopped. After another three days he was alright.

Case No. 110
INFLAMMATION OF TONSILS AND TONGUE

Dr. V. Sharma aged about 35, reported about his troubles of mouth. He was also running fever (100^0 - 102^0). On examination I found:—

(1)   His tongue was white coated.

(2)   Tonsils-enlarged and swollen.

(3)   Soreness in throat.

Further (i) there was no thirst, (ii) Difficulty in (a) swallowing even water and (b) respiration, and (iii) < motion.

I was aware of the fact that bio-chemic medicine could also be transmitted in the same way as Homoeopathic ones. Hence in this case, kali mur 12 x was transmitted (by dissolving 1 tablet of K.M. 12x in 1 dram of water, placing hair of the patient in the above solution and giving 10 strokes to the medicine phial).

E.T. (1)   Change in temperature of head was noted.

(2)   After 12 hours definite amelioration was reported.

(3)   After 24 hours there was no fever, no respiratory trouble and swallowing of food and drink was much easier. Tonsils were very little swollen.

(4)   After 48 hours the patient was free from all the troubles.

Hence transmission was made off after 72 hours.

Case No. 111
PAIN

My son, Madanjee aged 6 years was weeping on bed in the evening due to intense pain in his tongue. I found his tongue (1) Swollen, (2) Full of blisters and (3) Salivating. He was unable to take his meal, specially salty things. Besides this, watery discharge was coming out from his nose. As there was aggravation in the night, M.S. 30 was transmitted.

E.T. (1) Temperature of hand decreased within 1 mt.

(2)   Relief reported after 15-20mts. now the boy was not weeping, he was intending to sleep.

(3)   After 12 hours(next morning) he was much better, took his breakfast, reported very slight pain, tongue-better.

(4)   After 24 hours he was alright but transmission was still continued to study the further effect of transmission.

(5)   After 4 days, one morning he was continuously vomiting and suffering from headache hence transmission was stopped at 9 A.M. Again vomited at about 11 A.M., undigested food came out, intense vomiting tendency on waking, unbearable headache, occasional coughing and slight temperature(99^0-100^0) forced me to transmit Ipec. 30 at 11-15 A.M. after detaching from M.S.

(6)   Again vomiting at 3 P.M. and 7 P.M. very small amount of water came out.

(7)   In the same evening, he was better, but headache was still there, temperature was 99^0, at 8 P.M. he was given very small amount of diluted cow's milk.

(8)   In the next morning at 4 A.M. he again vomited, negligible small amount of water came out, after that he was alright, he ate, played, but very little headache was still left that day.

Next-day he was free from all the troubles but transmission of Ipec. 30 was still continued to study further effect.

(9)   After two days one night the boy reported intense earache, he was restless. It was the night of Diwali. Before that the boy fully enjoyed the various explosives usually made at Diwali night along with his friends. Someone said that these explosives caused earache. However, transmission of Ipecac.30 was stopped, within five mts.. the boy again smiled and played with his friends. In the night, he said to his mother "I feel as if my ear is vomiting". From the next morning he was perfectly alright.

Case No. 112
FEVER

My son, Kanhaiya jee aged 8 years was suffering from fever. Slight thirst, chill, intense headache < touch > pressure.

Cough was very prominent in this case. His liver region was painful as found on examination and also he was unable to sleep by pressing it. There was no pain on spleen side. Temperature was 101^0 at 11 A.M. China 30 was transmitted instantaneously.

E.T. 1. Rise in temperature of hand (r) was detected.

2. That day temperature went up to 104^0 (3 P.M.) & again began to fall. By 9 P.M. it was 101^0.

3. Next day in the morning(8.30 A.M.) temperature was 97.5, but at 10 A.M. it again rose to 100^0 & by 1 P.M. it was 101^0. Hence his symptoms were reviewed carefully and found marked change in the symptoms.

(a) Passed 4 stools - nothing characteristic was observed.

(b) Face white

(c) pupils of eyes dilated.

(d) Mind-Irritable.

(e) pain in the neighborhood of pit of stomach.

(f) Likes sweets.

(g) History of wetting bed.

Hence China 30 was detached & Cina 30 was transmitted at 2 P.M.

4. Fever at 9 P.M. 99^0 and 11 P.M.- 97.5^0 whole night temperature 97.5^0.

5. Next day alright, temp. 97.5^0 (whole day) hence he took his meal but transmission of Cina 200 was still continued.

6. After two days temperature of his body was observed to be 99^0 for only one hour (between 2 P.M. & 3 P.M) for two consecutive days only. Later on, he was alright, hence transmission of Cina-200 stopped.

Conclusion :-

On the basis of results observed in a number of cases, I am of the opinion that (a) Sahni's method of Transmission of Homoeo Drug energy from a distance is really a reliable method of patient.

(b) For cure of a patient correct remedy and potency both are required in this transmission method also.

(c) Period of transmission has to be varied from patient to patient depending upon his condition.

(d)   In case of aggravation usually transmission is stopped then amelioration starts rapidly, though this is not essential in all the cases.

(e)   Even after detachment and allowing sufficient time, if amelioration has not started, then another remedy must be transmitted according to symptom.

(f)   Bio-Chemic remedy can also be transmitted in a similar way as homoeopathic ones.

(g)   For speedy cure of a patient, a series of potencies of selected remedy may be transmitted according to requirements and detachment may be made from higher potency side in case of aggravation.

I expect that the Research Institute of Sahni Drug Transmission and Homoeopathy has taken up this project with encouraging results.

The author's remark :- (i)   Details about the project Series of potencies may be seen in the chapter on, "METHODS AND TECHNIQUE" and (ii) Regarding Transmission of Biochemic Medicines, the author's DRUG PICTURE OF BIO-CHEMISTRY" maybe read.

Case by **Dr. Lowry,**

501, Harding Avenue
William Sport, P A 17701
U.S.A.

Case No. 113
BOILS

(1)   "A 31 year old male named Mr. G. Singh was constantly suffering from boils in the nose and also on the buttocks and legs. After taking his full history, it was clear that he was a silicea patient in many ways. He came with me one day and insisted that I do something to get rid of the boils in his nose which were quite tender and inflamed. I told him I was going to try something new and asked for one of his beard's hairs. Upon explaining what I was about to do with the hair he became rather disturbed and said in many words what I was doing, was ridiculous and absurd and he did not believe in it at all. Just as he was continuing raving in this manner I placed the hair next

to the globule in the center fold of the Materia Medica. Instantaneously he said, "I feel so calm; Oh! this is ridiculous, it can't work". Within one minute he said that the pain in his nose was completely gone (he was as amazed as I was) then he said that there was another boil coming with pain and this subsided within one or two minutes. I was very impressed that his mental irritability vanished first and then the physical symptoms passed afterwards. This transmission was only kept for 5 minutes for it was very difficult to make sure the hair and globule were in contact with each other. This dose of Silicea 200 lasted for about 2 weeks until the boils returned again. Not understanding the method for liquid transmission which gives the case permanence to the treatment, I followed with an oral dose"

Case No. 114
COLIC

(2) "The other case was with another Sikh gentleman, Gurucharan Singh, 29 years old, suffering from a pain in his epigastrium which would allow him to eat only steamed vegetables and curd without pain. Being a rather irritable person and after taking his case, Nux-Vom. 200 was transmitted by the same globule method-relieving his acute pain immediately. Once again my ignorance of the new method forced me to give him an oral dose to complete the action".

THE AUTHOR'S REMARKS

(i) Dr. Lowry very frankly confesses her ignorance of the new method i.e. T.S. i.e. one dram phial containing solution of the selected drug along with the patient's hair. Thanks!

(ii) These experiments were made prior to her training in the Research Institute of Sahni Drug Transmission and Homoeopathy at Patna in India. After her training she is using the new method and she does not give any drug for oral use.

CHAPTER IX

VICTORY OVER TIME AND SPACE

It has already been stated that distance is no bar. Homoeopathic drug-energy can be transmitted to any corner of the world in no time. It may be transmitted even to the moon and other planets. In the first case of Transmission only a distance of five ft. was covered. The patient was sitting in a chair in front of the author's table. Gradually distance of 8,10, 300 feet, 228 and more than 500 K.M. was brought under the range of Transmission. Victory over space from Bihar to Jaipur,, Delhi, Amritsar and Bombay has been made in no time. Recently distance from Patna (India) to the U.S.A. has been covered in twinkling of an eye. Due to lack of communication difficulties are being faced. It needs a net-work of telephonic connections and the training of the public in large scale. In our country most of the people are away from telephone hence they may be deprived of quick effects of this discovery. The patients have to send letters by post and communicate the results in the same way. By doing so they have to suffer sometimes medicinal aggravation after transmission as it is not made off in time.

Sri J.P. Singh at Giridih sent his hair along with his symptoms. He had been suffering from whitlow in the middle finger of his right hand. Silicea 50 M. was transmitted on 12.12.1988 from Bettiah (Champaran) to Giridih. Slight aggravation in pain in witlow started from 12.12.68 and continued till 15.12.68. A letter from him was received on 30.12.68 that he was feeling better and transmission was on. On 21.1.69 a letter was received stating that his bowel was put in disorder with constipation and he had a violent toothache in the night of 15.1.69. The trouble was so intense that he was compelled by his family members to switch on to allopathy and take tablets, which he did very unwillingly but it also could not help much. Then the transmission was withdrawn at 11 A.M. on 21.1.69 and he was relieved. Sri Singh is a man of strong conviction and he could not have bowed down to that aggravation, had he known it to be medicinal, as he was not trained on the line of transmission for which the author is responsible. In this case the space-distance is about 500 K.M. and he was not available at phone. Had he informed timely he would not have suffered so much. It has been observed in experiences that in case of aggravation, the hair is detached from the medicine and the aggravation is checked. So long it is on, there is continuous flow of medicinal energy to the patients at distant places and during this period Hering's three laws-(i) From above downward, (ii) From within outward and (iii) In the reverse order of coming of symptoms, play their roles if the transmitted drug is selected according to the principle of "Similia Similibus Currenter". In case of Sri Singh the first law was working adversely.

Hairs of some Idiot and immovable patients from Ajmer and Jaipur were received along with letters which did not contain symptoms to arrive at the right remedies, hence Transmission was not done. The patients' guardians were asked to furnish detailed symptoms which could not be complied and they kept silent.

Mrs. Mehta of Jaipur, stating the condition of her daughter sent a letter, the extract of which runs as follows -

(१) लड़की की उम्र करीब ६ साल है।

(२) यह बोलने का प्रयास करती है पर बोल नहीं पाती है।

(३) इसे अत्यधिक हंसी आती है।

(४) यह नवीन व्यक्ति देखकर या कोई action देखकर इतनी हसती है कि काबू के बाहर हो जाती है।

(५) इसका मानसिक असंतुलन है और समझ में कुछ नहीं आता है। यहां के प्रसिद्ध डाक्टर का कथन है कि animal mind है। इसके हाथ-पैर सुचारू रूप से काम नहीं करते हैं। ऐसे तो चलती, भागती, खाती सभी कुछ करती है किन्तु लड़खड़ेपन से।

1. Her age is nine.

2. She tries to speak but could not.

3. She has immoderate laughing specially after seeing strange persons and actions, and gets beyond control.

4. She has no mental equilibrium. The doctor of great acumen of this place says that she has animal-mind.

5. Her limbs are not functioning well. She has staggering gait.

It may be observed that she is also a case of idiocy without detailed symptoms but there are some rubrics to arrive at some conclusions. The author was tempted to find out some remedy on whatever hints were there in the letter and transmit it. Hence on the following two rubrics only the case was repertorised according to "Kent's Repertory"-

(1)   Immoderate laughing :- **Am**. C., Can-i., Carb. V., Cupr., Ferr., Graph., Nat. Mur., Nux Vom., Stram., Stry., Tarent., and Zinc.

(2)   Idiocy - Nux-M.

Nux Moschata was selected and C.M. Potency of it was immediately transmitted on 22.4.1969 and a letter was posed to Mrs. Mehta, with some queries about further symptoms and effect of this Transmission. The report was received with the following extract on 23-5-1969.

(१)   बच्ची को हंसी में कुछ कमी अनुभव हो रही है।

(२)   बीच में छोटी माताजी निकल आयी थी जो २२-४-६९ से २९-४-६९ तक रही। फिर भी अब स्वस्थ है।

(३)   गत १५-२० दिनों से कागज व कोयला नहीं खा रही है जैसा कि पहले खाया करती थी।

(४)   सोने में एक अंगूठा मुँह में रखकर सोती है।

(५)   जाड़ा, गरमी का विशेष अनुभव नहीं है। कुछ कह तो सकती नहीं अन्दाज भी नहीं होता।

1.   Laughing is less now.

2.   Measles appeared on 22.4.69 and continued till 29.4.69. However, she is better now.

3.   She has not been eating coal or paper for the last 15 or 20 days as she used to take formerly.

4.   She sleeps with a thumb into her mouth.

5.   She has no clear conception of heat or coldness and moreover, she cannot express it.

Transmission of Nux-Moschata C.M. was kept on and further queries were made which were replied by her letter dated 28-5.69. The extracts run in the following way :-

(१)   इन दिनों पेट से दस्त के साथ निरन्तर कीड़े-बड़े-बड़े निकल रहे हैं।

(२)   पहले दस्त किसी भी जगह कर देती थी और मां का साथ जाना आवश्यक था। अब स्वयं फ्राक ऊँचा करके यथा स्थान पर बैठ जाती है।

(३)   इन दिनों गर्मी है, वह भी ज्यादा अनुभव करती है और पाँच-सात बार दिन में बाथ रूम में जाकर स्वयं नहा लेती है।

(४)   कमजोर व सफेदी लिये जा रही है।

(५)   खाना अलग रखने पर हमारे पास बैठकर अपने आप ही खा लेती है। क्या आप मेरे खर्च पर यहाँ आने की कृपा करेंगे?

1. These days she has been passing numerous big round worms with stools continuously.

2. Formerly she used to pass stool any where and she must be accompanied by her mother. Now lifting her frock high up, she passes stool at the proper place.

3. It is hot to-day and she also feels too much heat and she takes bath 5 or 7 times daily without any others help.

4. She is becoming weak and pale.

5. She, herself takes food sitting by my side if it be served separately.

    Will you please come over here at my cost?

Immediately transmission was set off on 2.6.1969 and he replied that his visit to Jaipur was not necessary then and it would be very expensive. Since then no response was made from her end and reason of which could not be learnt, and hence further information regarding effect of Transmission could not be gathered.

Dr. Raj of Bombay sent some hairs of a lady patient aged 25 on 26.5.1969 who had been suffering from mental derangement which was aggravated during change of seasons. The doctor was kind enough in diagnosing the case and informing that she was a patient of Nux. Vom. Hence immediately N.V. 50 M was transmitted on 29.5.69 at 12.20 P.M. A letter from Dr. Raj dated 6.6.1969 was received which reported that she had no trouble. Transmission was left on without any change in potency. Dr. Raj reported by his letter dated 8.7.69 that laziness had developed and she slept for 14 hours. Hence at once transmission was set off on 15.7.69 at 10.25 A.M.

A letter dated 4.8.69 from Dr. Raj was received wherein it was reported that she was just normal. Dr. Raj expressed his desire in the letter to pay a visit to his place at Bettiah, Champaran but he could not get there, though he was cordially invited in response to his last letter.

Dr. Raj sent hair of another patient suffering from Asthma. Symptoms were not sufficient to diagnose the case. Only nomenclature of the disease was there along with one hint that her mother died of cancer. Only only that history of cancer Carcinosin 50 M was transmitted but she could not be benefited. After this nothing was heard from his end.

204 Homoeo Drug Energy

One very responsible and experienced doctor of modern school of Therapy of Patna wrote on 18.6.69 :-

"Dear Dr. Sahani,

On hearing from my relatives that you are able to treat cases at a distance through the hair of the patient, I take this opportunity to take the advantage of the serious illness of my wife which is defying the modern medicine. She (age 50 years) is suffering from secondary metastasis in bones of pelvis, skull and other bones. She has a tumor also in the abdomen, a case of Carcinoma with secondaries in bones resulting in excruciating pain unrelieved by any known analysis and liabilities to fracture. She has finished irradiation with cobalt and Deep X'Ray therapy in bones. Nothing is left in modern medical science towards her care.

Hence, I am herewith enclosing a hair from her head for tele-treatment. If you happen to come over to Patna, please do intimate me so that I can personally see you about this case.

As a fellow practitioner in medicine I have every reason to believe that you will please take interest in the case of my wife. She is unable to move, sit, stand or turn side and all the time she is in great agonising pain with *Diabetes insipidus*. The diagnosis. of secondary cancer in bones is a confirmed reality. Hope this will not remain without drawing your personal attention.

Thanks,

Sincerely your's

'G"

Again the readers will see that there is not a single rubric except he nomenclature of the disease Cancer. Right remedy cannot be thought of for this case except Nosode-Carcinosin hence Carcinosin 10M was transmitted on 25.6.1969 at 7.15 A.M. and a letter expressing difficulty in diagnosing the case homoeopathically was addressed to him for symptoms in details in a short Case Taking Form. He was also requested to inform him on phone or telegraphically about the effect of this transmission especially in case of aggravation. Further he was requested to arrange a telephonic talk if possible but thereafter no response was received and the transmission was set off on 5.7.69. Reason for this silence could not be learnt.

Occasionally the author receives letters along with hairs

of patients from different parts of the country but due to paucity of symptoms transmission is not done and in case of hasty generalisation and transmission the result is not encouraging. This discovery being unique, people are not acquainted with its principles. In diagnosis homoeopathic principles are wholly taken into consideration. The chapters on "Treatment through Correspondence" and "Action and Duration" will make the readers acquainted with the method of treatment and its principles.

The author has already narrated that to cover time and space easy communication is essential. For this establishing hierarchy of Transmitting stations like Radio Broadcast system is needed. Main station may be established at the national head-quarter, Delhi or at Patna. Different sub-stations also may be established in remote parts of the country to transmit abroad. Co-opertion of Radio authorities is also needed to help in broadcasting programmes. etc. and educating people on this line to derive benefit from this cheap, easy and quick method of treatment without much botheration. The doctors practising in different parts of the country as well as abroad may extend their co-operation in experimenting this discovery and publishing the results. Many doctor friends practising in different parts of the country have been requested from time to time co-operate by sending hairs of patients along with their symptoms or names of remedies so that Transmission maybe done from our end, or by transmitting from their places through hairs sent by the author along with symptoms or names of remedies to cover time and space but no encouraging response has been received as yet. It would be his earnest request to the readers to think over this issue and extend their co-operation so that this discovery may prove a boon to the suffering humanity.

Even the so-called late acting remedies like Apis, Lycopodium etc. when transmitted act instantaneously at distant places. The examples of cure of urinary troubles of the heifer, Sri M. Singh and others in very short time are sufficient to justify this statement regarding Apis while the Prasad's example supports this regarding Lycopodium. Another example regarding victory over time is worth mentioning here. One tiny globule of Rhus Tox. 200 was sufficient to give quick relief to about 500 patients suffering from various ailments due to exposure to flood water in the flood affected areas of the Maner block, Patna in 1971. The peopele were surprised to see the results.

It would be interesting to mention here how this discovery spread to the U.S.A. and distance from India to America was covered. Miss Meredith Lowry of Wisconsin University, U.S.A. came across the author's book, "Transmission of Homoeo Drug Energy From a Distance" (Ist edition) and went through it. She experimented on some cases and was quite awed by the results. Hence she wished to study in detail and planned to come to India for Research in "History of Homoeopathy in India". She requested the author to give time and he agreed. She came to India and studied Homoeopathy. She also requested to undergo a course of training in the Research Institute of Sahni Drug Transmission and Homoeopathy. She was admitted into the Institute and she completed the full course of training. After completion, the fellowship of "THE RESEARCH INSTITUTE OF SAHNI DRUG TRANSMISSION AND HOMOEOPATHY" was conferred upon her. While she was in the Institute, she had some troubles. Her case history was recorded by the author and when she left India in the first week of June, 1977 and reached her country, Carcinosin 200 was transmitted through her hair without her knowledge on 5.6.77. It had immediate effect. Bleeding started profusely and she had temperature hence she informed the author on the cable on 11.6.77 at 5 A.M. when she had 104^0 temperature with profuse sweat. The hair was detached from the medicine and asked her to report soon. She promised to report next day. It has really a wonderful effect immediately after putting the T.S. off. Temperature came down after a few minutes to 102^0 and gradually it was normal and bleeding too was scanty by the next day. After some days bleeding stopped and she felt quite cheerful without any complaints. She had regular M.C. from the following month. In her letter dated 11.8.77 she has written "I wish to" tell that the bleeding ceased now for over one month and I had a very normal mense on this past full moon. "People of U.S.A. are amazed to hear this miraculous effect of Drug Transmission". Hence on the basis of this experiment as well as experiments shown in the chapter of "Experimental Observations" and others it can be rightly claimed that "Transmission of Drug Energy through the patient's hair from a distance" has got victory over time and space.

CHAPTER X

ACTION AND DURATION

Transmission of drug-energy is wholly based on the principle *Similia Similibus Curenter* of the father of Homoeopathy, Dr. S. Hahnemann. It is never a deviation. It differs only in method of application of drug to the patient. In the traditional Homoeopathic practice drugs are generally given orally. They are administered through olfactory as well as tactual organs also. This method of application may be called a direct method, i.e. drugs are directly administered to the organs. Transmission may be called an indirect method as there is no visual connection between the organ and the drug. It is just like Radio Broadcast System or wireless. Drugs in liquid, globules or in powder are brought in contact with a hair of the patient. They work instantaneously. In case of aggravation the hair is disconnected from the drug and more or less the action is checked. It awakens the vital principle which takes care of its domain. When the action of the drug exhausts it needs another jerk to maintain its energy to fight out the enemy-disease. Generally in practice one globule is dissolved in distilled or simple water in one dram phial and the hair by root is inserted into it and then it is well corked. There is continuous flow of energy from the phial to the patient. The patients get well day by day by this continuity, but sometimes there is aggravation after some hours, days, or weeks. Then Transmission is put off and drug energy once transmitted goes on acting till its expiry. Duration of drugs is counted from the detachment of the hair from the drug. Repetition, change of remedy or potency is made according to the strength of remedies. In the Organon Dr.Hahnemann has well described about repetition or change of remedy or potency. There are three rules to guide us in sticking to the first prescription. A remedy is never repeated when the patient is improving. In the same way Transmission is kept on so long there is improvement. It is never repeated when symptoms follow the Hering's three laws :-

(i)   From above downward,

208

Homoeo Drug Energy

(ii)   From within outward and

(iii)   Symptoms   appearing in the reverse order of coming. Remedy is also not changed when discharge or
eruptions follow the administration of a remedy.

It has been seen in one of the cases in chapter "Victory over
time and space" that the girl aged 9 of Jaipur had eruptions
(measles) just on the date of transmission of Nux Mos. C.M. and
since then she began to improve. In this case the Hering's 2nd
law was operative. The first law i.e. from above downward may
be observed in cases in chapter under the head "Experimental
Observations".

Mr. Prasad experimented the effect of Transmission of
Lyco. IM. firstly on his forehead-Tingling sensation with heat.
One minute after Lyco.200 was transmitted and he felt hot
sensation in his throat. Next time after one minute Lyco. 6 was
transmitted and perspiration from his palms vanished. Smil-
ingly the author asked Mr. Prasad which one was the right
remedy. He said, "The last one".

He was not acquainted with the principles of Homoeopathy, hence he replied in the above manner because perspiration
was also a headache for him. In the beginning of the discovery,
the author was zealous enough to experiment in all possible
ways. Hence sometimes he used to lose patience and make haste
in experiment. In case of Mr. Prasad, he could have waited for
a longer period. The last two effects might have been produced
by Lyco. I M but in hot haste he transmitted the last two
potencies one after another and hence confusion arose. These
days that hasty generalisation is not there in daily practice.
Once action starts in the right direction i.e. from above downward, Transmission is kept on to watch the further effects and
the percentage of success is better. Let us cite one example to
see how the third law of symptoms appearing in the reverse
orders acts. Mr. S. Prasad aged 24 of Muzaffarpur came to his in
the month of Dec. 1968. He had been suffering from Epileptic fits
from 1966 which was caused by suppression of eruptions by Nat.
Sulph 10 M administered by a homoeopath of great repute. He
was a sycotic patient (self acquired in 1962) and ill treated by
modern drugs. He was at a fix as to how to start, whether he
should antidote the effects of N.S. or give Medo. directly etc.
However, he repertorised the case and Stramonium 200 was
transmitted which had effect on his head. He was given the

transmitting set with him with sufficient placebo for a month.
While he was getting back home he had mild epileptic fit in the
carriage and the author was informed. He was ordered to
detach the hair from the phial containing Stramonium 200 and
he had been better that day. Next time Medo. C.M. was
transmitted and asthmatic trouble, which had started after
suppression of eruptions reappeared in spring of 1969 but he
had no epileptic attack. After some months Sulphur 0/5 was
transmitted and eruptions also reappeared. The patient discontinued the treatment. Medicines acted in the reverse order of
coming which is the Hering's third law. The readers will see
that all the principles of Homoeopathy are borne in mind while
selecting and transmitting drug-energy. Let us examine some
of the aphorisms and precepts of Kent also. According to Kent
there are three possibilities for second prescription :

(i) Repetition, (ii) Antidoting and (iii) Complementing.

Administration of a remedy as an intercurrent is not
favoured by the pure Kentian School. When a remedy is
administered to stir up or develop the case it amounts to
similimum and not an intercurrent and this view in Transmission is maintained. Sri H. Dubey aged 55 suffering from
laryngial cancer leaving all hopes to survive in spite of all
possible modern treatment, came to the author. His larynzial
growth was so big that it was impending respiration. The left
side parotid gland was very much enlarged and was hanging
below the left ear like an orange. His left cervical region was also
looking like a big lump. After diagnosing the case Lachesis 200
was transmitted and he got relief in respiration and swallowing
food without any reduction in size. Carcinosin 200 was transmitted after 5 weeks which was left on for a week and it was put
off when he felt some respiratory trouble, which vanished after
detachment of hair from the drug. There was a continuous flow
of Carcinosin energy for a week and then placebo was given for
a month. After a month Lachesis 1000 was transmitted (repeated) in the morning but in the evening there was aggravation in pain in his throat hence according to direction he
detached the hair from that phial and he got rid of pain. After
5 weeks the author was surprised to see the reduction in his
larynzial growth and placebo was given for another 10 weeks.
Then he felt pain in his throat and Lachesis 10000 was transmitted which gave him relief. After a week he got fever hence

Transmission was put off. Fever continued for a week and the parotid gland was reduced to normal size and cervical lump began to suppurate and he got alarmed as some doctors told that he would not survive if the lump would burst. The lump got open and copious thick yellow discharge began to flow. Gradually he felt better day by day and in a week the abscess healed up and he was very glad. The patient and the people were very hopeful and it was said that he was saved from the teeth of death, but misfortune was there in his store. He felt some respiratory trouble and Carcinosin 1000 was transmitted in the forenoon and was put off at 8 p.m. when there was aggravation in respiration. Placebo was given for a fortnight but respiratory trouble was not checked completely, hence he discontinued his treatment and switched on to modern treatment. This is how the transmission was repeated.

Dr. N.K.P. Sinha, who was transmitting Aconite 30 to Sweety, touched the remedy with the tips of his fingers and he got violent headache. He fainted, then the author transmitted Nux Vom. 30 to antidote the action of Aconite and instantaneously he got relief. During his practice he got very little change to antidote the administered remedies. Miss Sweety who got rid of Bcoli fever of one year standing after transmission of Aconite 30 and then Sulphur 30 was transmitted to perfect the cure which is a case of complementing a remedy. It has already been said that so long transmission is on there is continuous flow of energy to the patient. Let us clear this point by citing cases.

R.T. 200 was transmitted to Mrs. Pathak of Pathkouli, Champaran who had been suffering from gouty pain for many years. She immediately got some relief. The transmitting set (the phial containing R.T. 200 with her hair) was handed over to her with instructions to detach the hair from the phial in case of aggravation and sufficient placebo was given to take morning and evening. After a fortnight there was a violent aggravation in left toe and he had chance to see her at her home. He asked her where the phial was kept and immediately she replied, "Oh ! I forgot it. It is there in the box". On request it was brought to him and he put the transmission off and instantaneously pain vanished and again some placebo was given.

Mrs. Prasad aged 22 of Muzaffarpur had intense pain in her breast abscess. Carcinosin 200 was transmitted and the transmitting set was given to her to take home. The pain was tolerable. After two days her pain began to increase but transmission was not put off according to instruction. In the night pain was so violent that she became senseless and then it was made off but she could not revive her senses immediately. He had to go at 12 P.M. to see the patient but as soon as he got there she came to her senses. Placebo was given.

It has been stated in some cases in chapter under caption, "EXPERIMENTAL OBSERVATIONS" how the medicinal aggravation is checked. There are innumerable instances which go to prove the continuity of flow of medicine energy from the phial through hair to the patient. There are practitioners who practise transmission under his guidance, also on the basis of their experiences agree with the author that so long the transmission is on the action is continuous.

These days the transmitting sets are not handed over to patients as it was done previously.

The patients could not judge when T.S. should be put off. Sometimes they used to put it off when there was good action according to laws. In case of aggravation it is not essential to put it off in all cases. Aggravations take place and automatically they pass away in time. Some patients are careless and without putting it off they switch on to other physicians and their T. sets remain on for months together. In that case sometimes due to over-actions bad effects have been reported though some patients do not agree. Even if T. sets are kept in the author's chamber that danger is there. They do not care for transmission and switch on to other physician without informing the author. Once a high officer had been under the author's treatment. He continued it for some months but after transfer it was left on for about ten months. The author had chance to see him at his residence. He complained of tension in his mind and body with disturbance in sleep also. At once the author uttered that it might be due to the continued action of Drug Transmission, but he was unwilling to accept.

He ordered his son on telephone from his residence to detach hair from the medicine. No sooner it was put off, his tension vanished at once like magic. Since then he was very cautious of this transmission and once he, from bathroom asked his wife to request the author on phone to detach hair due to bleeding from anus.

If drug energy is transmitted for a second or minute to a patient, it stimulates the vital principle and goes on acting according to duration of that drug even after detaching the hair from the medicine. Hence in case of testing the remedies, or potencies the practitioners are doing much harm to the patients. Drug transmission is not a joke, it should be practised in the right perspective. However, the Homoeopathic principles and proving of various drugs are our real guide for action and duration in case of Drug Transmission also.

CHAPTER XI

TREATMENT THROUGH CORRESPONDENCE

There are three methods of treatment :

1.   *Personal interview* : Examination of the patient by the Physician. In this method the Physician himself collects signs and symptoms of the patients, their previous ailments, family history and other information by putting questions and cross-questions. The whole picture of the patient flashes before the Physician's mind. This is the best method of collecting data and treatment. On the basis of totality of symptoms medicine is selected and given to the patient orally or by transmission through detached hair or both by some of the author's disciples and followers (Pure transmission by the author).

2.   *Treatment through correspondence* : In this method the patients fill up the case taking form and send it to the Physician along with prescribed fees. The Physician on the basis of symptoms selects medicine and sends to the patient by parcel or prescribes the medicine to take orally. From time to time the patient sends progress reports and the Physician sends medicines with instructions accordingly.

In this case also medicine or prescription is sent with instruction to transmit it through detached hair of the patient's body. Generally one dram phial containing one dose of medicine (one globule) in distilled water is sent and the patient himself inserts one hair by root from his head into that phial and cork it tightly so that end of the hair may float in the air serving as an antenna. Direction is given to detach the hair from the phial in case of violent aggravation (of course intolerable) and ten strokes to be given to the phial to disperse sediments deposited around the hair and accelerate its action in case of *Stand-still-Condition.*

3.   Besides the methods mentioned above there is another method which is called by the author, *"TREATMENT THROUGH CORRESPONDENCE IN SPACE".* This is the

most unique and ultramodern method by which patients all over the globe can be benefited sitting in their sweet home by sending the case taking proforma duly filled in along with a hair from any part of the body, preferably from head and the requisite fees of the physicians. It would be better if a copy of recent photograph (full or passport size) is also sent. In this method everything is done by the physicians. Neither medicine is given orally nor it is sent by parcel to transmit or take orally. The Physician selects the remedy and transmits it through that hair of the patient, from his chamber on the 7th day from the date of dispatch of the hair, proforma etc. to any corner of India. In case of foreign countries like U.S.A., European countries, Japan or any corner of the World, drug energy is to be transmitted on the 15th day from the date of despatch of the proforma and hair. *Transmission* is generally done at 7 A.M. (Indian time) and patients concerned may observe actions and note them down from the 7th and 15th day from the date of dispatch respectively. They will generally send monthly progress report in the form attached in the end. If needed weekly or fortnightly reports also may be sent. In case of aggravation (of course intolerable) the physician should be informed by telephone, cable, wireless, telegram or letter so that he may do the needful. The patients having telephone facility are much benefitted by this method.

Patients from any corner of the globe may derive benefit. The patients should have firm belief in this method as this is most surprising and extraordinary. The patients by giving full history and symptoms along with hair, may be free from anxieties and cares of existing paraphernalia of treatment. They will be free not only from present ailments but also from the future ailments. The same hair may be used for all troubles to come. They will be free not only from present ailments but also from the future ailments. The same hair may be used for all troubles to come. The physicians in real sense of term will care, think and do the needful in their chamber on receipt of reports. This method is least expensive, easiest and quickest. As soon as the drug energy is transmitted, the patients at distant place experience the effect of drug in no time just like Radio Broadcast system.

GUIDE LINES

The patients as well as physicians should always keep in

mind that every case we take up is quite new and also that Homoeopathy treats the patient, never the disease by nomenclature. No doubt, nomenclature has its utility for communication but generally the people at large are haunted by its ghost hence they face difficulties in expressing the symptoms required by Homoeopathy. They do not distinguish between the symptoms of a patient and a disease. It has been observed that generally physicians and patients write down the names of their ailments in their letters and request for treatment, asserting that they are sending hair along with symptoms, but actually there is paucity of symptoms to select any remedy. It has been also observed that case taking form is not filled in properly. It may be either due to misunderstanding or due to non-clarity of rubrics in the form. One should not be puzzled to look at the exhaustive case taking proforma. This is meant for all ailments of humanity all over the world. He is to note only those points which concern him and the rest may be left blank. It should be noted that a well taken case is half done. Hence the proforma should be read again and again, and after due deliberation it should be filled in patiently. To know the individual patient his (1) *Mental symptoms,* (2) *Physical General*-Craving (strong likes) and aversions (strong dislikes) in food habit, (3) *Sex,* (4) *Sleep* and (5) *Generalities* (modalities-aggravations and ameliorations) of the patient as a whole are essential. These five are the structures out of which emerges the individuality of a patient. Throwing some light on these points will be helpful.

(1) *Mental Symptoms :*

These are divided under three categories-

(a)   Will,

(b)   Understanding and

(c)   Memory.

(a)   *Will* : All the instincts come under this head. All instincts are inborn hence no animals or human beings are devoid of them but there is a limit. Anger, fear etc. are normal. If any instinct crosses the limit of normalcy it is abnormal and taken into account for diagnosis. As for instance, *Anger*-Abusiveness, Cursing, destroying or throwing things, suicidal, tendency to bite, kill, pull hair, scratch body, tear clothes etc. in anger are abnormal behaviors on which Homoeopathic diagnosis may be based. In this way *Fear* may be considered. Every body is endowed with fear. Every one has fear of cobra, tiger etc. but when limit is crossed, it comes under the purview of symptoms. As for example, fear of dogs even puppies, cats, rats, other small animals, thunderstorm, water etc. is abnormal hence it is important for selection of a remedy. Every living being is gregarious and if it avoids society or has aversion to company, it is an abnormal behaviour for consideration. Any deviation from normalcy is abnormal and considered for diagnosis.

Every normal man has Sympathy but when he is cruel to creatures he is sick and needs treatment. Cruelity will be an important rubric for diagnosis. Sympathy too is considered when he is very sympathetic. Every rubric has three grades- much (Third), more (second) and most (first). While filling up the proforma (1st, 2nd and 3rd) must be noted against the rubrics so that accurate value may be attached in repertorizing. Every body *Weeps* but when one weeps and laughs alternately, weeps in anger, without cause, from joy, on past event, reading while, during sleep, in sympathy with others, telling sickness, when thanked, waking on etc. he is sick and *Weeping* will be a strong mental symptom for any ailment.

(b)   *Understanding* : delusions, illusions etc.

(c)   *Memory* : weak for what-name, place etc.

(2)   *Physical General* :

Generally people take rice, bread, fish, meat, eggs, milk, fat, curd, pickles, sweets, vegetables, fruits, salt etc. Mere likes or dislikes for these menu do not come under purview of symptoms. They are normal. Any deviation from the norms are the guiding symptoms which speak of the patient as a whole. If the non-vegetarian have developed aversion to fish, meat, eggs etc. and the vegetarian to milk, vegetables, sweets etc. for which they had liking previously; and they developed craving for any menu which they had disliked or mere likes, then those items of food are guiding symptoms, i.e. craving for cold food, fish, meat, milk, salty things, earth, coal, pencils sweets etc. or aversion to them. Any item taken swallowed or abstained against desire under the medical instructions are not to be considered. One may have craving for milk, sweets, fish etc. and by taking them his trouble aggravates, hence he abstains from taking them but while giving replies to such questions in the proforma if he notes down that he has no liking for those items then it will be a blunder and right remedy can't be selected. These will come under craving and aggravations by taking them will be noted in generalities. This type of vague reply is generally given by the patients and right answer is derived after cross-questions by the physicians but when the patients are away from the physician and they have to depened on the data in the proforma hence greater caution is needed. It is better to give no answer than giving wrong or confused answer.

(3) *Sex :*

The chapter on sex (Male & Female) has been dealt with as particular but it has got the importance of Physical general or Generalities. Aversion to coition (intercourse), enjoyment absent, no discharge during coition, violent sexual desire, masturbation, menses etc. speak of the patient as a whole hence greater care should be taken to fill it up. Frank dealing without concealing the fact counts much. Generally patients feel embarassed in answering such questions but without exactness and correctness of the rubrics in this chapter right diagnosis is not possible.

(4) *Sleep :*

It comes under general. Every body has got his own style of sleeping. Some will sleep on high or 2-3 pillows while others may not tolerate even low pillow. Some covers mouth and nose with clothes while others do not like to sleep even in a closed room. Some may sleep with one hand on head while another under it. One may prefer to sleep on back while other on sides. Some sleep like a dog or on knee-elbow positions while others on abdomen.

So is the case with dreams. Some have sleep with full of dreams while others have a little. Different dreams-horrible, amorous, pleasant etc. have their different symbols which are important hence names of the symbols (animal, death, snakes, stool, urine, marriage, eating etc.) must be given. Dreams are guided by unconscious mind-the depth of human mind, hence they reveal many suppressed desires and ambitions. Hence they are important along with sleepiness or sleeplessness etc.

(5) *Generalities :*

Last but not least, Generality plays a very vital role in diagnosis and it becomes a major premise when there is lack of mental symptoms or Physical generals (cravings or aversions to menu of food) hence it should be clearly understood and mentioned against each item of ailments as well as the patient as a whole under the following heads :

Modalities : Aggravation or Amelioration-(a) Exact time A.M. or P.M. if known, morning, in bed, waking on in night, rising after in morning etc.

Aggravation or Amelioration-(b) (i) before, during or after stool, bath, eating, fasting, intercourse, lying on, menses, sitting, standing, sleep, movements stooping etc.

(ii)   Winter, spring, summer, rainy or Autumn seasons.

(iii)   Heat or cold application, hot or cold food or drinks etc.

(iv)   Closed room, crowd, fan, moonlight, noises, sun etc.

If pain in abdomen or leg (particulars) be relieved by warm application, it does not mean that the patient as a whole also likes warmth or warm weather. He may like cold season, (general). His head pain (particular) may be relieved by washing with cold water, though the patient as a whole (general) is chilly. What is true of a particular organ may not be true of the whole person.

Particular modalities have been mentioned along with different organs and generalities which speak of the individual as a whole, have been noted in the last chapter. The above lines are the pegs against which the Homoeopathic diagnosis is hung and if they are weak or wrong, it will kiss the ground.

Besides the above lines, causation or aetiology is of paramount importance and has got a vito power. When it plays its role, it becomes major permise and the above mentioned ones become minor premises. As for example, unconsciousness, grief or love-disappointed, abuse of quinine, epilepsy after onanism (masturbation), T.B., asthma etc. after suppression of skin diseases etc. Hence causation should never be missed while filling the proforma up.

Once more it is cautioned that answer should be given after due deliberation and never in a hurry. The wrong or confused answer will lead to wrong selection of a remedy which will be harmful to the patients as well as the physicians.

If the patient has difficulty in filling up the proforma, he may take help from a good local Homoeopath.

The history of the patient is to be given in the following proforma :

1. (a) Name :
    (b) Age :
    (c) Caste :
    (d) Occupation :
    (e) Full address :
    (f) Phone :

2. Present troubles with dates or years :

3. Previous past ailments suffered from :

    Treatment - (Ayurvedic, Allopathic, Homoeopathic) with results. (T.B., Itches, Ringworm, Eczema, Pneumonia, Malaria, injury by fall or accident, Bites-dog, snake and insect, warts, shock, masturbation, syphilis, Gono. etc.)

4. Pathological test :
    (a) Previous, if any.
    (b) Recent, if any.

    (Blood, Urine, X-Ray Report, E.S.R., W.R., V.D.L.R., Electro-cardiogram, Biopsy etc., if any with dates).

5. Family history :
    (a) Father :
    (b) Mother :
    (c) Brother and sister (dead and alive) :
    (d) Marriage-date with year :
    (e) Wife or Husband and
    (Children (dead and alive).

    Note : Ailments suffering or suffered from, general health etc.

6. If any family member suffers or suffered from Cancer, T.B., Asthma, Diabetes, Syphilis, Gonorrhoea, Mental trouble, Leprosy, Warts, Malaria and use of quinine, Eczema and other skin diseases.

    Note : Maternal and paternal sides, duration of illness treatment and years.

7.   Mind :
     Educational qualifications with Classes or Divisions.

     (a)   Will : Anger, Irritation, Fear, Suicidal tendency,
           Miser or Extravagant, Talkative or Taciturn, Hopeful
           or Despair of recovery, Sympathy, Reaction to
           consolation, Disappointment, likes-loneliness or
           company, if weeping why-in anger, hearing music,
           telling symptoms etc.

     (b)   Understanding :
           Illusions, Delusions and Hallucinations. Any fixed
           ideas etc.

     (c)   Memory :
           Weak for what-name, place etc. Lost-Past or Recent
           events etc.

8.   Sensorium : Vertigo, Giddiness-with aggravation and
     amelioration, time etc.

9.   Head : Condition of hair, falling, gray, dandruff, curly,
     headache-time, Aggravation and Amelioration, High
     Medium or Low pillow, whole or one sided pain, sweat etc.

10. Eyes : General condition - Vision :

11. Ears : General condition - Hearing :

12. Nose : Epistaxis, cough and cold, sneezing, Adenoids,
     polypus, any other growth, snoring, smell, picking or
     itching etc.

13. Face : Sunken, Greasy or Dry, Eruptions etc.

14. Mouth : Aphthae, blisters, bleeding, smell, taste, salivation,
     tongue-colour, dry or wet etc.

15. Teeth : General condition, pyorrhoea, caries, Extraction,
     loose, pain with aggravation and amelioration etc.

16. Throat :

     (a)   External-Goiter, glands, swelling etc. thick or thin.

     (b)   Internal-Dry, Tonsils-sides-swallowing difficulty in
           liquid, solid or empty. Lump objective or subjective,
           pain etc. Aggravation by cold or hot application etc.

17. Stomach :

     (a)   Appetite-more, normal, less or loss.

     (b)   Craving-Liking for milk (cold or warm), sweets,

salty things (salt more, normal or less), meat, fish, earth, ice cream, coal, cold or hot food, sour things, bread and fat food etc.

(c)   Aversion (Dislikes) to Acids (Sour things) bread, fats and rich food, cold or hot food, meat, milk, salty food, sweets, smoking, water (cold or hot) etc.

(d)   Thirst : Thirstless, with dry or wet mouth. Thirst-normal, extreme-quantity number of times and taste etc.

(e)   Nausea and Vomiting, if any-when-morning, while brushing mouth, before, during or after eating, during sleep etc. pain with time, aggravation and amelioration etc.

Note :   General condition, better before or after eating, Mere likes or dislikes are no points, hence caution is to be taken to fill up this column.

18.   Abdomen : Condition of liver and spleen

Likes loose or tight clothes-Distension, Dropsy, Flatulence, Fullness, pain-time and modalities-Aggravation and Amelioration, Rumbling, Sensation of something alive or movement - Swelling, Tension etc.

19.   Rectum and stool :

Constipation, Diarrhoea-time with Aggravation and Amelioration, constriction, Haemorrhoids-bleeding or blind-Colour of blood; Nature of pain with aggravation and amelioration, involuntary stool-while coughing, laughing, sneezing, passing flatus or urine.

Itching : when, polypi or any growth, prolapsus-when before, during or after stool or passing urine etc.

Stricture, swelling, any sensation of lump, weight etc., worms etc.

Stool-colour, balls, long, dry, loose, thin, watery, etc.

(a)   Bladder-Constriction, sensation of fullness, inflammation, pain with time and modalities. Retension of urine, urging-constant, frequent, ineffectual, dribbling, feeble, divided stream, Involuntary, Bed-wetting, while-blowing nose, during coughing, passing flatus, laughing, lifting, sitting, walking, sneezing etc.

(b)   Kidney-Heaviness, Inflammation, pain with modalities etc.

(c)   Prostrate Gland - Emission, Enlargement, Inflammation, pain etc.

(d)   Urethra - Constriction, crawling sensation, Discharge, colour, Gonorrhoeal, thick or thin, Haemorrhage, itching, pain before, during or after urination or constant etc. Stricutre, swelling, tingling, or twitching sensations etc.

(e)   Urine-Albuminous, Alkaline, Bloody, Burning-when-before, during or after urination, colour, copious or scanty, milky, smell, sediment, specific gravity, sugar, thick or watery etc.

21.   Genitalia :

(a)   Male - penis relaxed, absent sensation, cold or normal, when more painful, eruptions, falling of hair, involuntary handling. Hydroceles-sides-Inflammation, itching, crablice. Disposition to masturbation-when-pain with modalities, sweat, phimosis or paraphimosis, seminal discharge-bloody, copious, difficult, failing during intercourse, incomplete, late, painful and quick.

Seminal emission-nightly, interval, with or without dreams, involuntary, before, during or after urination.

Sexual passion-Less, more, excessive. violent, wanting or normal.

Smelling, Tingling sensation, tumor, twitching, ulcers, warts etc.

(b)   Female-Abortion-how-fright or injury after, which month. Abscess, aphthae etc.

Cancer-uterus, cervix, vagina.

Coition-Aversion, enjoyment absent, late discharge or absent.

Desire-less, more, violent, driving to masturbation.

Displacement of uterus, eruptions, itching before, during or after menses, heat, inflammation.

Leucorrhoea-acid, bloody, copious, colour, more before, during or after menses, offensive, during pregnancy, thick or thin, colour.

Masturbation-Menopause.

Menses-absent, colour, copious, first menses delayed, frequent, intermittent, late, offensive, painful, last date and duration of menses.

Pain - Ovaries, uterus, vagina, during intercourse. Prolapsus-lifting, menses before, during or after, during stool, passing flatus etc.

Sterility-Swollen, tumors, warts etc.

22. Larynx, Trachea, Respiration, Cough, Expectoration-Trouble, time of aggravation and amelioration, modalities-sitting-, walking, sleeping, lying on sides   back, L., Rt., on abdomen, cold, hot, colour-thick or thin etc.

23. Chest-Tightness, Haemorrhage, Inflammation, Breasts-Lump, Milk-bloody, absent, in non-pregnant; in boys etc., oppression, pain with modalities, paralysis, sweat, T.B., Heart-palpitation with modalities, Lungs etc.

24. Pulse - Regular, rapid, full, thready, intermittent.

25. Back-Abscess, Burning, coldness, curvature, eruptions, abnormal sensation, heaviness, pain with modalities and locations, stiffness, twitching, tumors, weakness etc.

26. Extremities :

    Abscess, Arthritis, Awkward gait, Brittle nails, Burning, Caries of bones, chorea (Trembling), coldness, constriction, cramps, crippled nails, deformities, discolouration, eruptions, ematiation, heaviness, incordination, inflammation, ingrowing nails, itching, lameness, lightness feeling, numbness, pain-nature, location and modalities-better by motion, cold, heat, worse by motion, cold, heat etc. Habit of shaking limbs (fidgety), stiffness, swelling, tension, tingling, twitching, ulcers, warts, weakness, wooden sensation etc.

27. Sleep :

    (a) Deep, disturbed-which part of night, restless, sleeplessness.

    (b) Dreams-Accidents, anxious, coition, danger, dead body or person, eating, drinking, falling, fire, flying, ghosts, marriage, money, murder, nightmare (walking during), quarrel, robbers, thief, snake, snake-bite, urine, stool, storms, suicide, water, weeping etc.

(c)   Position : On abdomen, arms over or under head, on back, crossed limbs, limbs drawn up or apart, on knees and elbows.

Sides - L. or Rt., sitting etc.

(d)   Sleepiness-when, yawning etc.

Pillow-without, low, medium, high or two.

28.   Fever :   Chill or shivering, heat, sweat, thirst, number and quantity. Time. Other accompanying symptoms like nausea, vomiting, headache, pain etc.

29.   Skin :   Anaesthesia, Biting, Burning, Cancer, Coldness, cracks, discolouration, dryness, Eruptions, Formication (abnormal sensation), Greasy, Itching, Lump, Sweat-on which part mostly, colour of stain of sweat on cloth, lousiness and when, swelling, ulcers, warts, wrinkles etc.

30.   Generalities : Modalities :

(a)   Better by day, forenoon, noon, morning, evening, night etc., cold, heat, sitting, walking, lying down on which sides, standing, spring, summer, rainy season, autumn, winter, food and drink-which one before, during and after eating, menses, and bath, dread of bath, open air etc.

(b)   Worse by - what and how ?

All the above columns are to be filled in carefully otherwise right remedy cannot be arrived at. The serial numbers 3, 5, 7, 17 (specially likes and dislikes), 21, 27 and 30 are the pillars on which the edifice of diagnosis is constructed, hence they should be filled in very carefully. Vague answers should not be given. In case of confusion, straight replies in "Do not know or Do not remember" should be given.

After filling up this case taking form properly, it along with one or two hairs from the head, or any organ should be sent to the doctor, who will transmit the rightly selected remedy on the fixed time and date. In case of aggravation, the doctor should be informed immediately by Telegram, Telephone or Express letter, so that he may put the transmission off to check the aggravation and do the needful. The readers will now realise the author's difficulties, which he has been facing due to paucity of symptoms given by the patients without knowing the principles of Homoeopathy which treats the patient and never the disease.

WEEKLY/FORTNIGHTLY/MONTHLY REPORT

Ref. No.................

Date   Period

1. Description of each ailment pointing out differences :

2. Reappearance of previous ailments with date and period from............to.............

3. Change if any in mental symptoms pointing out differences......

4. Change in physical generals....carvings....aversions....

5. Change in Generalities or other modalities....

6. Weight

7. The points which were left in filling up the proforma if any —

8. Difference in health on the whole....

CHAPTER XII

MERITS OF TRANSMISSION

In every sphere man has been striving to reach perfection. From bullock carts to rockets ? What a wonder ? Science today is doing miracles. It has got victory over time and space. Journey to moon has been made possible. Many more advancements are to be done in future which cannot be apprehended at present.

Medical Science is also trying its best to go ahead. Heart is planted. Eyes are planted. No wonder ! A time may come when it can produce man without man and woman. No doubt it has expanded in length and breadth but time and space have not been conquered though doctors in foreign countries can examine and control patients from a distance particularly in heart diseases. Homoeopathic Science is trying to expand in volume and depth but now by discovery of "Transmission of drug-energy through patient's hair" it has got victory over time and space. Its one more dimension i.e., height has been expanded.

In medical therapy other that Homoeopathic therapy drugs have got physical properties subject to chemical laws, but Hahnemann, the father of Homoeopathy has proved that potentized medicines "are no longer subject to chemical laws". Further it has been added that "a powder of Phosphorus in highest potency may remain for years in its paper in a desk, without losing its medicinal properties, or even changing them for those of Phosphoric Acid". Homoeopathic drugs are dynamic hence they are transmissible. Some of my doctor friends of modern school have tried to transmit their drugs specially Belladona in colic but they have not been successful so far. The author has personally no experience if medicines of other schools can be transmitted or not.

1.   The first and foremost importance of this discovery is that it proves supremacy of Homoeopathy over other pathies inasmuch as no other drug than Homoeopathic is transmissible so far.

2. It has got victory over time and space because the reaction through "Transmission" is instantaneous and it is not necessary that a patient should be before the doctor at the time of transmission. A distance from Bihar (India) to Jaipur, U.S.A. etc. has been covered so far. The girl patient's hair from Jaipur was sent in an envelope along with her symptoms. Nux Mosch. C.M. was transmitted from Bettiah, Champaran, Bihar and she was influenced by the drug-energy there at Jaipur the very same day. The Chapter on "Experimental Observations" may be re-examined for other cases. Recently a girl patient of the United States of America has been treated successfully in no time.

3. The reaction through "Transmission" is immediate in case of almost every medicine including Lycopodium, Apis etc. which are said to be slow in action. It is said that Lycopodium reveals its action in a week or 21 days but the author does not know how this notion has been formed. Even in oral method it is not found true. No doubt, this drug is deep-acting and acts for a longer period but it is not a fact that it remains inactive for days together before manifestation of its action in a week or so. It may be that the practitioners could not detect its action earlier and they formed this notion. Even during proving Lycopodium has shown its action in two minutes after its administration. In the same way Apis is said to be slow but with a qualification of "sometimes". It may be in this case also that the action might not have been observed earlier. Dr. William Boericke in his book, "Pocket Manual of Homoeopathic Materia Medica" says "sometimes action is slow, so several days elapse before it is seen to act......" In experience it has been observed that Apis 30 has acted instantaneously when transmitted. Sri M. Singh of Champaran, a very chronic case of urinary trouble who had been carrying a bottle fitted with a rubber tube to his bladder to collect urine, whose urinary passage was permanently blocked by stricture in spite of all miraculous drugs and several operations costing about a lac, had been under his treatment. He had improved very much and the bottle and tube had been thrown. One day he had pain in his penis with retension of urine. Apis 30 was transmitted to him who passed urine immediately and was free from

pain. Transmission can drive out that notion of slow action from the minds of its holders.

4. The flights of Apollo 11 and 12 were controlled from the earth without any visible connection. The driver controls the vehicles by a steering or a break. The players control the flights of kites in the sky, of course through threads in their hands but there is direct (not wireless) connection in these cases.

In the field of medical therapy once a drug is administered there is no control over its action. In case of aggravation either it is antidoted or checked by other drugs to the detrimental effect on the economy. Transmission has supremacy over other pathies and oral method of Homoeopathy in this direction also. It is easier to control the aggravation of any medicine transmitted through hair. Here the doctor is only to switch it off i.e. he has only to detach the hair from the medicine and aggravation is checked immediately. It has been seen how Sri Mandal, Mrs. M. Kumar and others in "Experimental Observations" and Mrs. Pathak under "Action and Duration" have been given relief by putting the transmission off. In case of wrong action of a drug also transmission antidotes and gives relief to the patient. Dr. N.K.P. Sinha who was transmitting Aconite 30 to Sweety, mentioned under "Experimental Observations" was affected resulting in blind headache and Nux Vom. 30 was transmitted by him and he got quick relief.

5. In modern medical therapy urine is cultured to test the sensitivity to drugs in case of B-coli infection and then the drug which is sensitive is administered to check the disease. In Homoeopathic field sometimes diagnosis, i.e. selection of right remedy becomes difficult and drugs one after another are administered wasting time and producing drug diseases, but in transmission medicines can be put to test in a few minutes and arriving at the right one it can be transmitted. This trial and error method is never to be encouraged. One must labour to select a right remedy and then transmit. However, transmission has got some merits in saving time.

6. Selection of potency of Homoeopathic drug is a great problem in practice. Potency in Homoeopathic therapy is

unique and peculiar. There is a great hierarchy of potencies from mother tincture to C.M., C.M.M. etc. It can be said that potency is just like soul in a body. It is very difficult to find its existence out with the aid of mightiest modern instrument or machine except by experience. Its selection is an arduous task. Different practitioners use different potencies in their practice. Some are high and medium while others are low potenists. Dr. Kent was a high potenist and his followers also follow him. Dr. William Boericke along with others was a low potenist. In the beginning of practice the standard of using potencies is not established. It is established only by experience though the school to which one belongs modifies the standard.

"Transmission" helps the practitioners in selection of potencies also. It has been observed in one case under "Experimental Observations" how Lyco 1 M, 200 and 6 were transmitted to Mr. Prasad and Lyco 1 M was finally selected. As soon as the "Transmission" is on, effect is felt in disposition-mind, head, eyes, ears, nose, face, mouth, throat, chest, heart, abdomen, extremities or skin etc. as mentioned in the chapter "Mechanism of Transmission" and so with help of Hering's three laws - (i) From above downward, (ii) From within outward and (iii) In the reverse order of appearance of symptoms, right potency may be selected without wasting any more time. Hence it saves time also.

7. The patients have to undergo ordeals during the course of treatment. The modern medical therapy has cumbersome paraphernalia through which they have to pass. They are dragged from place to place and have to spend a lot over their journey etc. Day by day treatment is getting costlier. Transmission has come to help the ailing humanity without any paraphernalia and botheration. Treatment through transmission is the cheapest of all. It is economical to the patients as well as to the practitioners. The patient may remit the reasonable amount fixed by the practitioners and send one hair with his or her symptoms. The rest will be done by the doctors and he or she will enjoy treatment sitting in his or her sweet home. The practitioners have to spend a very little quantity of medicines. Even one

globule saturated with potentized drug may be transmitted to a number of patients if a little care is taken. Once the author had chance to serve and treat about 500 patients with a single globule of Rhus Tox. 200 dissolved into ordinary water in the Maner Village of Patna during the flood of 1971. The people from the flood affected areas were brought in boats to Maner in rescue measure and they took shelter in schools or community halls. Most of them were indisposed having temperature, headache, backaches, lumbago, pain in body etc. due to exposure to flood water for days together hence R.T. was selected as an appropriate remedy. One dram phial-solution of one globule of R.T. 200 was divided into 4 phials and kept at 4 centres. They were advised to insert hairs of different patients into those 4 phials and whenever they were empty, they were refilled with fresh water and some strokes were given. In this way most of them got relief in no time.

8. The method of transmission is very handy and simple in comparison to other techniques so far invented in the field of therapy. Handling of Emanometer, Radiesthesia, acupuncture, Zone therapy, the Science of Cosmic Rays therapy etc. are very cumbersome. Transmission can be done anywhere very easily.

9. Some practitioners and the people in general have been deluded by one of the age-long misconceptions that Homoeopathic medicines are not effective to the smokers, betel chewers with tobacco etc. Smoking, zerda, smell etc. neutralise the actions of drugs, hence they are reluctant to come to us for treatment. Many are firm believers that Homoeopathy will never cure them because they smoke. They are not at fault. The idea has been filtered down to them from us that is why they hold this misconception. Wherefrom this misconception has sprung ? Perhaps it has sprung from maintenance of purity at the time of provings as well as in practice. During provings of drugs all the exciting factors are removed so that they may not confuse the actions of drugs. Suppose a subject during proving of a drug takes zerda (tobacco) and gets giddy. Confusion arises if this giddiness has been produced by tobacco or the drug. Hence purity is strictly maintained

and it must be maintained in practice also but not at the cost of science itself. This misconception is a stigma on the part of Homoeopathic science that actions of the subtle medicines will be neutralised by smoking, smell etc. There are some practitioners who are not ready to take up the patients addicted to smoking or tobacco in any form. There are others who advise them to maintain many rituals (many do'ts) during treatment. No doubt, smoking is detrimental to health but habit being the second nature of man is not easily shuned. Hence one must be considerate otherwise he will lose more.

Let us cite a few instances as to how the potentized drugs act even while smoking or chewing betel with tobacco. Once Thuja 10 M was given to a Civil Surgeon who was smoking at Dhanbad and one engineer who was sitting by his side in his chamber spoke out, "He is smoking". The author promptly replied, "What of that ! It is not so tender to be neutralised by smoking. If it be so then there are many things in our system which may neutralise it". The Civil Surgeon supported him and he took it with benefit. An officer at Hazaribagh, suffering from intolerable pain in his rectum due to haemorrhoids got instantaneous relief though he was chewing betel with tobacco. Formerly he asked for a glass of water to clean his mouth but he told if he had the belief that medicine would not act while chewing betel then he would not be allowed to clean it. A tiny globule saturated with medicine was given in his hand to put it into his mouth. He kept the betel in one side of his mouth and the globule in another side. The belief that the betel saturated with tobacco would spoil the action of the medicine was still lurking in his mind like ghost in spite of his sermons but after relief he realised the reality. Innumerable cases have been treated successfully in this way only to remove the misconception.

It is true that exciting factors must be removed from the way in course of treatment as far as practicable but not at this cost. The subtle potentized similimum will not be neutralised by the gross-smoke or smell. It does not mean that he does not believe in antidotes.

The method of "Transmission" is enough to wipe out the age-long-stigma stamped on the Homoeopathic therapy. Those, who never thought to undergo treatment in the hands of

Homoeopaths due to their smoking habits now come to those who practise "Transmission" saying that this discovery has come only for them (the smokers, chewers of betel with tobacco etc.) because they have not to take medicines orally. They believe now that smoking will not spoil the action. Some practitioners following "Transmission" also have begun to shun that misconception. A time may come when that misconception will completely be removed from the minds of the people and the practitioners holding that, and thus both will be benefitted.

10. "The Discovery of Drug Transmission" opens a vast field for further researches on its different aspects like Radiations from hair and human body, Relation between separated hair and the body. Potencies and space, Relation between separated poison and scorpion or snake. Mundan (Ritual shaving of a child for the first time) and hair, (why to put hair in a sacred place ?), Electronic Energy and Potency and Spiritualism, "Kirlian aura" and radiation from T.S. etc. Besides these it may lead to other discoveries in the different disciplines of science.

11. Last but not the least Drug Transmission is advantageous not only to the patients and practitioners in removing its above stigma but it also contributes to the science of Homoeopathy. Homoeopathic science has already reached the fathomless depth and has been expanding in length and breadth. The discovery of Transmission has added the fourth dimension, i.e. height to it and it has supremacy over other pathies. It is evolving like an organism.

Human mind by nature is very conservative. It is not ready to believe what is not perceived by its own eyes. Though seeing is believing still sometimes it hesitates to believe even after having personal experience. That is why even the intelligentia class show apathy and are not prepared to believe in "Transmission of drug-energy through patient's hair". Sri Sinha, a man of high calibre, mentioned in the Chapter on the "Experimental Observations", who was bed-ridden due to sciatic pain, got rid of his trouble by Transmission; and still he suspected if Transmission had actually worked. Many others also who were benefited had doubt to believe it. What is talk of others ? Even today there are people who do not believe the working of Radio system and space science is beyond their comprehension. Discovery is never at fault, if it is beyond their conception. Space science once upon a time an imagined faction now has turned out to be a reality !

CAUTION : Transmission of drug energy influences the patient immediately and deeply. Merits Nos. 5 and 6 are being misused inspite of caution given on pages 101 and 102 of this book (the first edition). If one drug is transmitted on the patient it has its effect on him and if perchance that is not the similimum, another drug is tried and in this way many drugs are tried. Every drug has its own effect on the patient and thus all drugs producing their bad effects, make the subject complicated and incurable by producing drug-diseases. It is seen that some miraculous effects are exhibited to catch the attention of people for the time being but in the long run it proves ineffective. Hence some followers of this method are causing immense harm to the patients by using this sacred method as a Radiesthesia only. Instead of a boon, it may prove a curse to the suffering humanity if this practice is adopted. This weapon must be used according to the principles and one should always bear in mind the words of Dr. Kent that the Homoeopathic failures are the worst failure on earth. One should labour hard to find out the similimum to bring the disordered economy in order. Hence the author once more humbly draws the attention of his followers (of this method of Drug Transmission) that bombardment of many dynamic as well as crude drugs should not be done on the innocent patients and it should not be used as a Radiesthesia only.

BIBLIOGRAPHY

1. Dr. Boericke, G.M. : (1063) "A lipoid test for the selection of Homoeopathic medicine" Torch of Homo. 5(3)-165.

2. Dr. Hahnemann S. : (1955) Organon of Medicine translated by R.N. Dudgeon and comments by B.K. Sarkar, M. Bhattacharya Co., Cal.

3. Dr. Hanshaw, G.R. : (1966) "Laboratory Experiences with Homoeopathic remedies" Jour. Met. Ins. 55 (9-10) 296-99.

4. Dr. Hobbs J.A. : (1961) "Radiesthesia and Radionic Diagnosis" Torch of Hom. 3(4) 236.

5. Dr. Sahni, B. : (1967) "Homoeopathic Dynamic Medicine can be transmitted" Torch Hom (2) 93-95.

6. Dr. Prakash, C. : (1967) Ibid. Editorial notes.

7. Dr. Moitra, S.K. : (1967) "The Mysterious potencies" Torch of Hom. 9(2).

8. Mitra S.K. " "An introduction to the Philosophy of Shri Aurobindo".

9. Chatterjee, S.C. and Dutta, D.M. : "An Introduction to Indian Philosophy".

10. : Navneet 'Hindi' Digest Page 21 of August, 1967..

Under : -Khoj-Khabar.

"Bal bhi Nar aur Mada".

"Hair too,male and female".

11. Dr. T. Sinha : "Medical Radiesthesia".

12. Dr. B. Bhattacharya : "The Science of Cosmic Rays Therapy".

13. Dr. S. Seal : "Research In Homoeopathy In India".

14. Dr. B.N. Saxena   : "The Torch of Homoeopathy" Jan. 1961, page 45 to 48.

"The Dynamic action of Drugs and Plants by their external exhibition from Distance".

15. Dr. Chandra Prakash   : Editorial notes on......do.....

16. Dr. P. Sankaran   : "Some Recent Research and Advances in Homoeopathy".

17. Dr. Wethered, Vernow   : "An Introduction to Medical Radiesthesia and Radionics".

18. Dr. Gray   : "Anatomy".

19. Dr. Banerjee, P.N.   : "Chronic Diseases".

20. T.F. Allen, A.M., M.D.   : "The Encyclopedia of PURE MATERIA MEDICA" Vols. I and VI.

21. J. Bernard Hutton   : "HEARING HANDS" - "A strange, true adventure in Psychic Surgery". "Fascinating" - Library Journal Introduction by Dr. E.T. Bailey, M.B.B.S., F.R.C.S.

22. Robert H. Thouless   : "Experimental Psychial Research.

23. L.E. Eeman   : "Co-operative Healing"

24. Hering's Domestic Physician

25. Dr. Shrinivas   : (Main Kahan Hoon).

26. Kent.   : "Lesser Writings".

27. Kent.   : "Philosophy".

28. Kent.   : "Repertory".

29. Hering.   : "Guiding Symptoms" Vols. VI and VII.

30. Gentry   : "Concordance Repertory Vol. VI".

31. Tyler   : "Drug Picture".

32. Dr. Morton Whitby.   : "Theory of life, Disease and Death", quoted by Dr. Seal.

33. Dr. Otto Lesser M.D.,   : "Critique of Homoeopathy".

Ph.D

34. "Wright"   : "Applied Physiology" quoted by
                                  Dr. S. Seal.

35. "H.C. Jones"   : "Theory of Electrolytic Disso-
                                  ciation", quoted by Dr. S. Seal.

36. T.H. Mc. Gavack, M.D.   : "The Homoeopathic Principles
    Head of the Department   in Therapeutics" quoted by
    of Homoeopathy,   Dr. Seal.
    University of California
    Medical School.

37. B.S. Bahl and G.D. Tuli   : "Essentials of Physical
                                  Chemistry".

38. B.R. Puri, M.Sc., Ph.D.   : "Principles of Physical
    F.R.I.C. (London) and   Chemistry".
    L.R. Sharma M.Sc. Ph.D.

39. Samuel Glasstone,   : Text Book of Physical
    D.Sc., Ph.D.   Chemistry.

40. Prof. S.N. Mukherjee,   : "Introduction to Physical
    D.Sc.   Chemistry" Vol III (Advanced).

41. Peter Tompkings and   : "The Secret Life of Plants".
    Christopher Bird.

42. Akhand Jyoti   : Sep. _1972 (Pages 25-27)

43. Stuart Close   : "The Genius of Homoeopathy".

44. S. Hahnemann   : "Chronic Disease" Part I.

45. Kent.   : "NEW Remedies".

46. "Akhand Jyoti"   : September, 1972.

47. F.K. Bellokossy,   : "There are no Medicines" The
    M.D. Colorado.   Hahnemannian Cleanings Vol.
                                  XLIV, No. 4 April, 1977.

48. Yoga   : Thought and Practice. Fifth
                                  anniversary, 1974-Indian In-
                                  stitute of Yoga.

49. Yoga   : "Pranic Mind Field". June 1977,
                                  Bihar School of Yoga, Monghyr,
                                  by Swami Satyamurti Sarswati,
                                  Ph. D., N. Ireland.

50. WHM Fitz Geald, M.D.   : "Zone Therapy"

& Edwin F. Bowers M.D.
51. Dr. Eric H.W. Stiefvater : What is Acupuncture ?
and Leslieo, Korth, D.O.
M.R.O.
52. Sonya Richmond   : "Yoga and your Health".
53. Dr. B. Sahni   : "Case Taking proforma with guide lines".
54. Stanley Kripper and   : "The Kirlian Aura"
Daniel Rubin.   "Photographing the Galaxies of Life".
55. Dr. J. Kishore   : "Card Repertory".